Save a Life

The ABCs of CPR

Barbara W. Trefz
American Heart Association
Basic Life Support Instructor

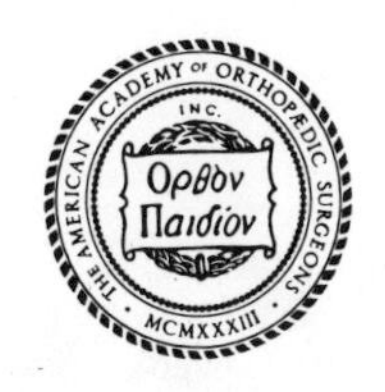

American Academy
of Orthopaedic Surgeons

The material presented in this book has been made available by the American Academy of Orthopaedic Surgeons for educational purposes only. The material is not intended to represent the only, or necessarily best, methods or procedures for the medical situations discussed, but rather is intended to present an approach, view, statement, or opinion of the author(s) or producer(s) which may be helpful to others who face similar situations.

Printed in the United States of America

ISBN 0-89203-026-7

Many of the illustrations found in this book were reproduced with permission from *Emergency Care and Transportation of the Sick and Injured,* ed 4. American Academy of Orthopaedic Surgeons: Park Ridge, Ill., 1987.

TABLE OF CONTENTS

SECTION 5: UPPER AIRWAY OBSTRUCTION IN INFANTS AND CHILDREN

SECTION 6: PROFESSIONAL RESCUER/HEALTH CARE PROVIDER SUPPLEMENT

ACKNOWLEDGMENTS

This booklet is based on materials found in the following publications:

1. "Standards and Guidelines for Cardiopulmonary Resuscitation (CPR) and Emergency Cardiac Care (ECC)," published in the Journal of The American Medical Association, Vol. 255, No. 21, June 6, 1986.
2. Instructor's Manual for Basic Life Support, American Heart Association, 1985.
3. Instructor's Manual; Totsaver, American Heart Association, Westchester/Putnam Chapter, Inc., undated.
4. "Tips to Make Child's Summer Accident Free," Wisconsin State Journal, June 9, 1986, N.Y. Times News Service.
5. "Stress—Friend or Foe?" Wisconsin Division of Health EMS Newsletter, Vol. 7, No. 1, November 1985.
6. "Movement of the Patient Who has Suffered a Cardiac Arrest." Joe Ketarkus, RN, Madison General Hospital, Madison, Wisconsin, undated.
7. Emergency Care, Barbara W. Trefz, EMS Coordinator, Methodist Hospital, Madison, Wisconsin, 1982.
8. Emergency Care and Transportation of the Sick and Injured, 4th ed., American Academy of Orthopaedic Surgeons: Park Ridge, Ill., 1987.

With special thanks to:

- Joe Topp, AHA-BLS Instructor, for permission to use S.T.O.P. for discontinuing CPR.
- Judith A. Johnson, RN, AHA-BLS Affiliate Faculty, for early review and comments.
- Bob Napolitano, Pat Becker and Harold Farkus, for their support and encouragement.
- The many concerned professionals associated with the 1985 National Conference on Cardiopulmonary Resuscitation (CPR) and Emergency Cardiac Care (ECC).

INTRODUCTION

At 10:35 on a warm summer night, the people leaving the Orpheum Theater witnessed a brutal fist fight between two young men. One of them received a severe blow to his stomach and fell with a thud to the sidewalk, unconscious. The stunned crowd stood silently. Not one person came forward to aid the injured man. A feeling of helplessness came over me. A voice within me shouted—"Do something!—Somebody Help!"

Perhaps you, too, have witnessed a situation where you knew something should be done but were at a loss as to what to do. Perhaps you know someone who has already experienced a medical crisis, and may need your help in the future. Perhaps you are taking this course to fulfill a job or school requirement. No matter what the reason, it's comforting to know that the information you read in this booklet, in combination with the training you receive in class, will give you the skills to help out in a medical emergency.

This booklet is divided into six sections. Section 1 contains the following general information:

- Selected facts and figures
- Methods for accessing emergency medical services
- Safety and legal concerns
- Overviews of the cardiovascular and respiratory systems
- Hints for healthy living/recognizing risk factors
- Hints for recognizing and managing specific medical emergencies.

Sections 2–6 are divided into adult and pediatric training modules and contain supplemental information for health care providers and professional rescuers.

CERTIFICATION

A prerequisite of CPR certification is enrollment in a course taught by instructors affiliated with the American Red Cross or the American Heart Association. Successful completion of an authorized course requires that the student pass written and skill performance tests. This booklet provides the reader with appropriate information; however, skill practice and written and practical testing must be provided by and take place in the presence of an authorized instructor.

SECTION 1: GENERAL INFORMATION

SELECTED FACTS AND FIGURES

In 1981, over 3,000 deaths in the United States occurred because food or other items lodged in a person's airway. Objects stuck in the mouth and throat can obstruct the airway, bring about unconsciousness, and, if not corrected, lead to cardiac arrest—a condition in which the heart stops beating.

Each year 350,000 Americans die of cardiac arrest before they reach a hospital. *Cardiopulmonary resuscitation (CPR)* is a technique that combines rescue breathing and chest compressions in an attempt to restore respiration and circulation. Recent studies from communities that have offered training to large numbers of people document that more than 20 to 30 percent of people who suffer out-of-hospital cardiac arrest can be saved! Two factors account for this success: (1) immediate citizen CPR and (2) prompt advanced life support care by ambulance and hospital personnel.

CPR is *basic life support,* which means that it requires no special equipment, just proper training. *Advanced life support,* however, requires additional training in drug administration, the use of machines for monitoring heartbeat, the insertion of tubes to maintain an open airway, and mechanical devices to provide ventilation.

ACCESSING EMERGENCY MEDICAL SERVICES

The initial help given a victim is the first step in a well-organized system of emergency care. This system includes citizens, emergency communicators/dispatchers, first responders (police, firefighters, rescue squads), ambulance and hospital employees. Today, specially trained and licensed personnel reach the ill and injured in sophisticated land, air, and water ambulances. Nearly all areas of the United States are serviced by emergency medical service systems.

An *emergency medical service (EMS)* system provides more than transportation. The system is made up of separate components linked in a special way for the purpose of providing emergency medical care. The system works this way:

1. The citizen discovers the ill or injured person, provides initial care, and calls the emergency dispatcher. If ambulance service is not available, the citizen arranges transportation for the patient to the nearest hospital providing 24-hour emergency care.
2. First responders and ambulance personnel arrive, give further care, and transport the patient to the hospital.
3. Hospital employees reassess the ill or injured person and provide definitive treatment.

Gaining access to emergency medical care can be as simple as dialing 9-1-1 on your telephone to contact the emergency dispatcher. Unfortunately, this universal emergency telephone number is not available in all communities. Local emergency telephone numbers are usually listed on the inside cover of telephone directories. Since emergency numbers are rarely posted near telephones you should memorize the appropriate numbers to call from your home and at work. Avoid dialing "O" (operator). The operator may not answer right away or worse yet may connect you with a telephone operator in another state, thus causing a delay in contacting local responders.

After reaching the emergency dispatcher, give the following information:

1. Location of incident (address, cross streets, mile markers, or prominent landmarks).
2. Number of people needing attention.
3. Type of problem(s) needing action.
4. Condition of victim(s).
5. Care presently being given to victim(s).
6. Additional help needed (police, fire).
7. The telephone number, including area code, from which you are calling.

To make certain the dispatcher has all the necessary information, *hang up last.*

HEALTH AND LEGAL CONCERNS

Certain safety and legal considerations should be examined before you begin training.

Safe Training

This course will bring you into close contact with training manikins. Although over 40 million people have been trained in CPR, there are no documented cases of bacterial, fungal, or viral diseases caused by manikin use. The issue of cross-infection is less of a threat if people who have any type of illness observe the following warning from the American Heart Association:

No student can participate in manikin training who has:

1. sores on the hands, lips, or face.
2. a known positive hepatitis surface antigen (hepatitis).
3. an upper respiratory infection such as a cold.
4. AIDS (Acquired Immune Deficiency Syndrome).
5. a current active infection or recent exposure to an infectious source.

(Instructors Manual for Basic Life Support, A.H.A., 1985.)

Proper sanitizing techniques are observed with manikin practice. Your instructor will outline decontamination methods.

This course does include some physical activity and emotional stress. If you have questions regarding your ability to take this training, please consult your personal physician.

Legal Considerations

Many states have "Good Samaritan" laws that provide an exemption from civil liability for people who help in an emergency. To date, no one who has performed CPR reasonably has been successfully sued.

If you are a public safety official whose job description requires medical response or if you are a citizen trained in emergency medical procedures, you should do the following:

1. Start action by providing care for the ill or injured person, and notifying the emergency dispatcher.
2. Continue care until the person revives, another trained rescuer takes over, a physician or physician-directed person or team takes over, or you are too exhausted to continue.

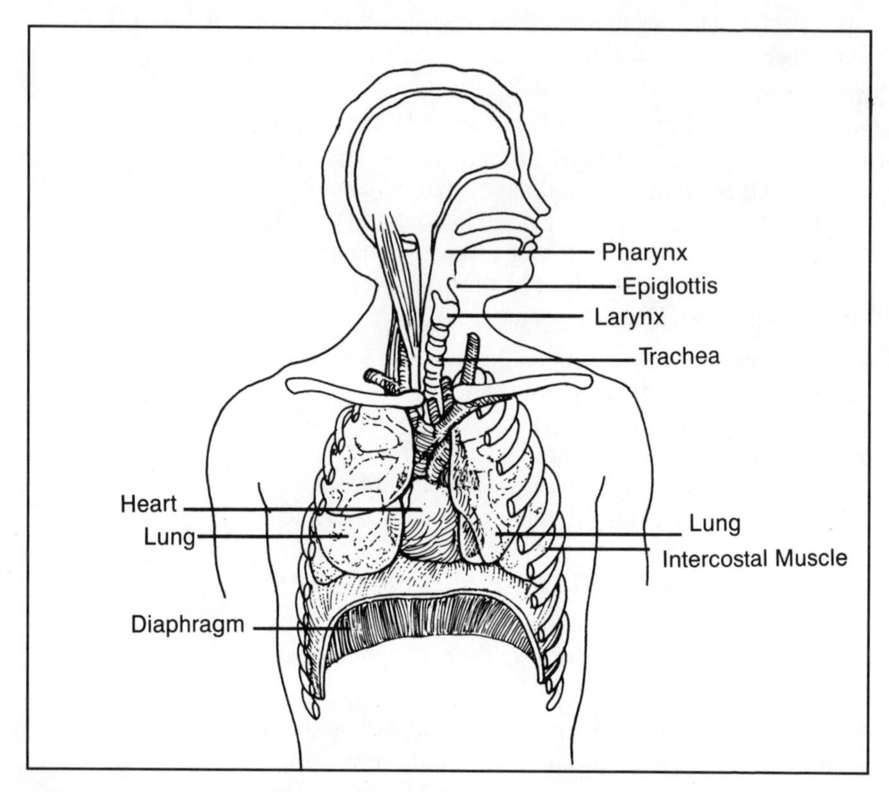

Figure 1
Location of the heart in the chest cavity.

No action should be taken if the person is truly beyond help and exhibits any of the following signs of death:

1. Decapitation
2. Tissue decomposition
3. Dependent lividity (black and blue on areas where the body has rested)
4. True rigormortis (the stiffness seen in corpses)

It is important to point out that victims exposed to cold may appear to have rigormortis. However, start CPR because there is mounting evidence that these victims can be saved with CPR.

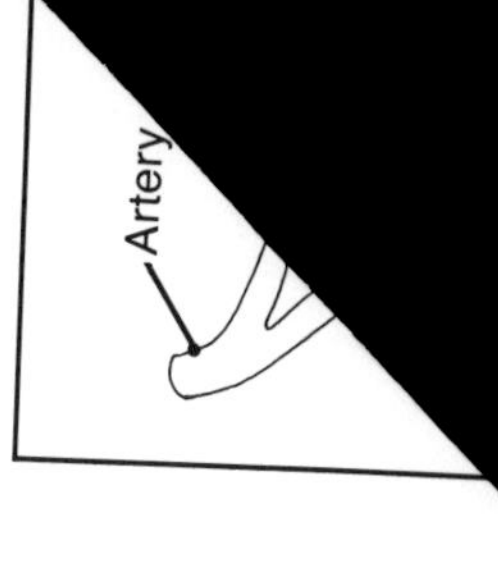

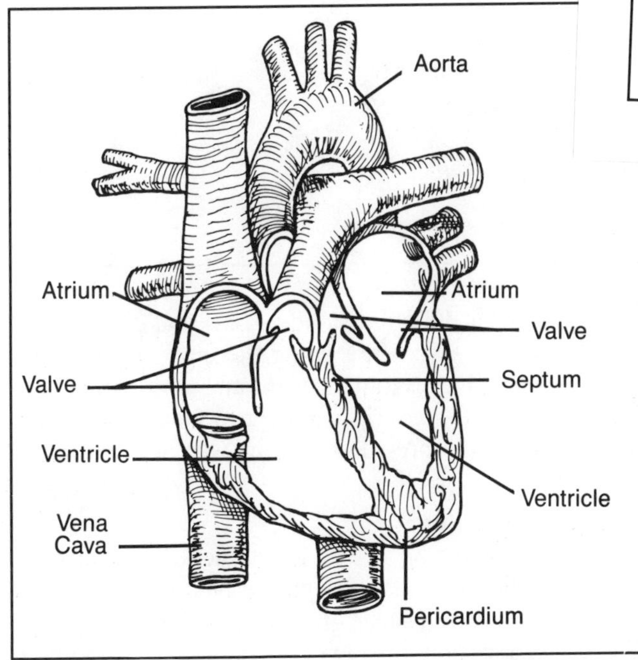

Figure 2
Structures of the heart.

THE CARDIOVASCULAR AND RESPIRATORY SYSTEMS

This course deals with recognizing and correcting life-threatening problems in the cardiovascular and respiratory systems. An overview of these systems serves to clarify emergency action procedures and helps emphasize that maintaining a healthy lifestyle and minimizing risk factors can prevent certain medical emergencies.

Cardiovascular Structures

The cardiovascular system consists of the heart and three types of blood vessels (arteries, veins, and capillaries). The heart is a muscular, fist-sized organ located within the chest between the lungs and behind the breastbone (sternum). (Fig. 1) The outside of the heart is covered by a protective sac called the pericardium. Inside the heart are four chambers (atria and ventricles) which are divided lengthwise by a wall called the septum. One-way valves separate the atria and the ventricles. These valves direct the flow of blood within and from the heart. (Fig. 2) Arter-

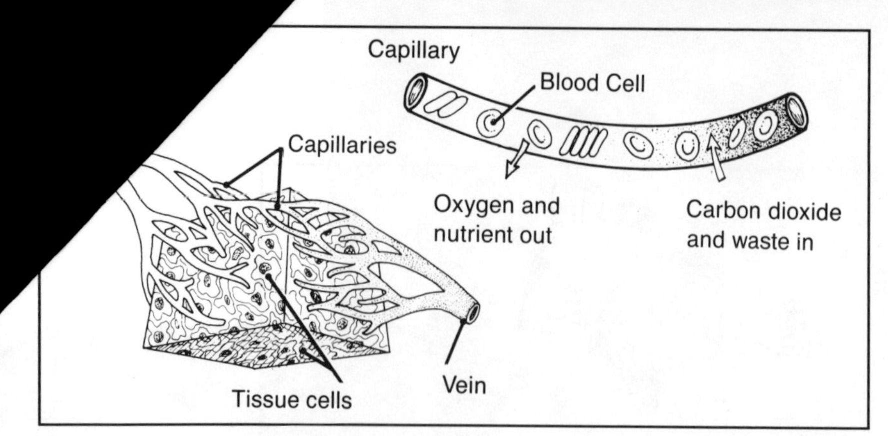

Figure 3
Specialized vessels carry blood to all parts of the body.

ies are muscular, tubelike blood vessels that carry blood away from the heart. Veins bring the blood back to the heart. Tiny capillaries join the veins and arteries and provide blood to all tissues. (Fig. 3) Special vessels (coronary arteries and veins) provide the heart with its own blood supply.

Cardiovascular Functions

The function of the heart is to pump blood carrying oxygen and carbon dioxide through the blood vessels to all parts of the body. Exchange of oxygen (which is needed by all cells) and carbon dioxide (a waste product), occurs in the capillaries. Oxygen enters and carbon dioxide exits the body through the lungs.

Both sides of the heart pump simultaneously. Veins bring oxygen-depleted blood into the right side of the heart through the vena cava. The right ventricle pushes the blood to the lungs where carbon dioxide is given off and a fresh supply of oxygen is obtained. The left side of the heart receives the oxygen-rich blood from the lungs and pumps it through the body's largest artery (the aorta) to all parts of the body. Pumping action is initiated by specialized electrical impulses generated within the heart. This action can be measured by locating a pulse and counting the number of beats per minute. Pulse sites are found where arteries lie close to the skin's surface (for example, the neck, arm and wrist). Adults at rest average 60 to 80 pulse beats per minute, although well-conditioned athletes may have a much lower rate. Infants and children have

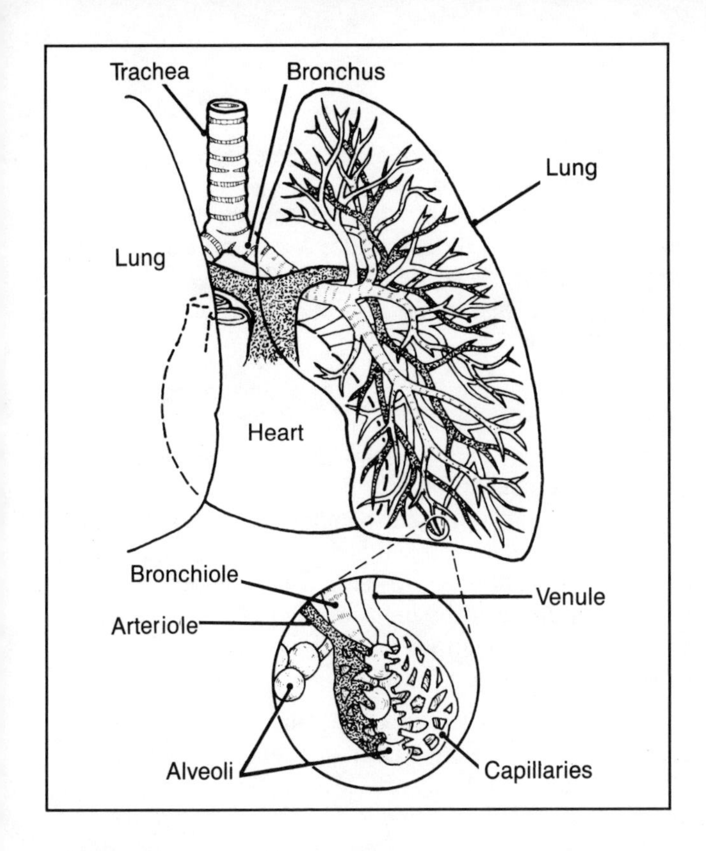

Figure 4
The Respiratory System.
Figure 5
Structures of the lower airway.

higher pulse rates. For example, newborns average more than 100 beats per minute, and seven-year-olds average 80 beats per minute.

Respiratory Structures

The respiratory system is divided into upper and lower airways and include all structures that receive the flow of atmospheric air into the body. (Fig. 4)

The upper airway consists of the nose, mouth, pharynx (The space behind the tongue), and the voice box (larynx). When a person swallows a flap of tissue (the epiglottis) covers the larynx to keep foreign materials out of the lower airway.

The lower airway contains the windpipe (trachea), two extensions called bronchi that branch from the trachea into each lung, multiple smaller branches called bronchioles, and the alveoli. Alveoli are tiny grapelike clusters of air sacs that are surrounded by capillaries and make up the spongy part of each lung. (Fig. 5)

Respiratory Functions

The function of the respiratory system is to bring in oxygen and push out carbon dioxide. A continuous supply of oxygenated blood is needed by every body cell. If something happens to disrupt the flow of oxygenated blood, cell death will occur.

Breathing is an automatic process. Adults at rest breathe approximately 12 times a minute, infants, 20 times a minute, and children, 15 times a minute. Special sensors in the brain send signals to the muscles of respiration; the diaphragm, a thick dome-shaped membrane located below the lungs, and the intercostal muscles found between each rib. As the diaphragm and intercostal muscles contract, the ribs lift upward, the lungs expand, and air rushes in. This is called inhalation. Exhalation occurs when these muscles relax and air is pushed out.

Atmospheric air at sea level contains approximately 21 percent oxygen, 79 percent nitrogen, and trace amounts of other gases. The body absorbs less than one-quarter of the oxygen taken into the lungs. When air is exhaled, the ribs and diaphragm relax and the unused oxygen, carbon dioxide, and other gases are released. Since the body uses only 5 percent of available oxygen, this released air, combined with rescue breathing techniques, contains enough oxygen to support the life of a person who is not breathing.

HEALTHY LIVING

The cardiovascular and respiratory systems are interdependent that is, they cannot function without each other. That is why it makes sense to promote a life-style which limits risks to these systems. Studies have shown that people who control their weight, eat sensibly, exercise regularly, and avoid smoking are less likely to encounter problems with their cardiovascular and respiratory systems.

Weight Control

Adults reach their optimal weight in their early twenties. As time goes by, people tend to eat as much but exercise less and the result is the storage of extra calories in body fat. Proper control calls for judging the amount of food needed to maintain correct body weight. Your personal physician is the best source for health-related information. After evaluating your age, weight, build, and medical history, your physician will make suggestions for any necessary changes.

Sensible Eating

Our bodies function best when fueled by balanced meals consisting of foods selected from the four food groups: milk, meat, fruits/vegetables, and grains. Six other measures contribute to sensible eating:

1. *Avoid salt/sodium and foods containing large amounts of sodium.* Salt contributes to high blood pressure (hypertension), so limit its use in cooking and at the table.
2. *Avoid saturated fats and cholesterol.* Saturated fat and cholesterol cause a buildup of fatty deposits in the arteries. Saturated fats are found in certain vegetable oils (palm, coconut, heavily hydrogenated margarines, and shortenings); dairy products (whole milk, cream, butter, ice cream, and cheese); and bakery goods. Cholesterol is present in egg yolks, organ meats, shrimp, and lobster.
3. *Limit eggs.* Since egg yolks contain cholesterol, eat three or fewer yolks each week.
4. *Select polyunsaturated fats.* A sensible diet includes the use of polyunsaturated fats which act to lower blood cholesterol levels. Polyunsaturated fats are found in vegetable oils and polyunsaturated, nonhydrogenated shortenings; and corn, soybean, and safflower products.
5. *Select fish and poultry.* Four to six-ounce portions of fish or poultry should be eaten more frequently than other meats. When choosing meat, pick lean cuts.

6. *Select skimmed milk products.* Check labels for percentage of fat present in dairy products. Lower fat levels are preferable.

Regular Exercise

Exercise tones muscles, stimulates circulation, aids weight control, reduces stress, and makes us feel better. An active life-style that incorporates activities to increase heart rate (e.g., brisk walking, climbing stairs, running, cycling), performed 15 to 30 minutes every other day, can prevent heart disease. Your physician should be consulted before starting an exercise program. Although exercise is essential for physical fitness, strenuous or unaccustomed activities may bring on a heart attack in the person with undiagnosed heart disease.

RECOGNIZING RISK FACTORS

Weight control, sensible eating, and regular exercise are ways to encourage cardiovascular and respiratory fitness. Other elements contribute to good health. Some of these can be controlled; others cannot.

Risk Factors That Can Be Changed

1. *Smoking.*

   The facts are in on smoking, and the news is not good. The following facts sum up the bad news:

   a. Smoking can initiate and add to the buildup of fat deposits in arteries.
   b. Smoking is the most important single cause of preventable death in the United States.
   c. Cigarette smokers experience 70 percent more coronary heart disease than nonsmokers.
   d. Smokers are two to four times as likely to face sudden death. The more you smoke, the greater the risk.
   e. For women taking oral contraceptives, smoking increases the risk of heart attack.
   f. For women who smoke as much as men, the risk of coronary heart disease is similar to men.
   g. Smokers have a greater risk of dying from a variety of other diseases.

There is some good news, however:

a. People who stop smoking have a lower death rate from heart attack than smokers.

b. After a period of years of abstaining, the death rate from heart attack will be similar to that of non-smokers.

c. Lung tissue damaged by smoking will gradually improve-if smoking is stopped.

If you are a smoker, consult your physician. There are programs specifically designed to help you STOP. If you are a nonsmoker, don't start!

2. *Obesity.* Consult your physician. There are programs specifically designed to help you reach your proper weight.
3. *High blood pressure* (hypertension). High blood pressure is symptomless; however, stroke and heart attack can result if hypertension goes undetected. A blood pressure reading of 160/95 is considered hypertensive. Mild hypertension can be treated by reducing weight and limiting salt (sodium) intake. If these methods do not succeed, your physician will prescribe antihypertensive drugs. Since there are no short-time cures for hypertension, management of this risk factor is a life-time commitment.
4. *Blood cholesterol levels.* To avoid the buildup of fatty deposits in the inner walls of blood vessels, follow a diet low in saturated fats and cholesterol. Sometimes medications are prescribed to lower blood serum cholesterol levels.
5. *Diabetes.* In people with diabetes, a deficiency of insulin prevents the body from using glucose (sugar) as an energy source. Diabetes often appears during the middle years and is dangerous because it greatly increases the risk of heart attack. In the diabetic, all risk factors must be carefully managed. If you experience the following signs and symptoms, consult your physician for evaluation and treatment. Signs and

symptoms of diabetes can be very subtle and easily attributed to other problems:

a. frequent urination
b. extreme thirst
c. constant hunger
d. weight loss or gain
e. weakness or fatigue
f. blurred vision
g. slow healing of cuts, scratches
h. numbness in hands or feet

6. *Stress.* Stress has been described as "the rate of wear and tear within the body." Stress occurs as a physical or psychological response to crisis. Physical reactions include increased heart and breathing rates, nausea, chills, and excessive sweating. Psychological or emotional reactions include anxiety, excitability, and apathy. Not all stress is bad. Moderate stress provides motivation—gets us ready to act. However, heavy stress can produce long-term physical and psychological pressures. If emotional or physical symptoms warrant, consult your physician for help with stress management.

Risk Factors That Cannot Be Changed

1. *Heredity.* In families with a history of early heart disease, this tendency may be an inherited factor.
2. *Sex.* Men have a higher incidence of heart disease. However, the risk for women greatly increases in postmenopausal years, most likely because the drop in estrogen allows a buildup of deposits in arteries.
3. *Race.* High blood pressure is found more often in blacks.
4. *Age.* The death rate from heart disease increases as we age, yet one in four deaths from heart disease occur before age 65.

By modifying risk factors and promoting a healthy lifestyle, we are less likely to encounter problems with the cardiovascular and respiratory systems. Medical problems such as atherosclerosis, angina pectoris, heart attack and the many causes of sudden death occur when the body does not receive enough oxygenated blood to maintain normal functioning.

Atherosclerosis

Atherosclerosis is caused by a buildup of fatty deposits in the arteries. These narrowed passageways increase blood pressure — that is: the pressure of the circulatory blood against the walls of the arteries. As the blood pressure rises, the heart has to work harder.

When blood pressure is measured, the first number recorded is the *systolic pressure,* which is the pressure within the arteries when the heart contracts (beats). The second number recorded is the *diastolic pressure*, which is the pressure within the arteries when the heart relaxes (between beats). With atherosclerosis, diastolic pressure is often above 90 mm Hg. (millimeters of mercury).

Emergency Management of Atherosclerosis: Consult a physician for specific programs and medications.

Angina Pectoris

Angina pectoris is characterized by pain in the chest, neck, jaw, and shoulder or arm brought on by any activity that increases heart rate and blood pressure. Angina is usually the result of atherosclerotic buildup in the coronary arteries — the arteries that feed the heart.

Emergency Management of Angina Pectoris: Rest and/or nitroglycerin (a prescribed medication) should relieve symptoms within 10 minutes. If pain persists, this may indicate heart attack. Follow emergency management procedures for heart attack.

Heart Attack

Heart attack (acute myocardial infarction) occurs when severe narrowing or blocking of a coronary artery prevents bloodflow to a portion of the heart muscle (myocardium). The affected part dies, which disturbs cardiac pumping and creates abnormal electrical rhythms. Heart attack can happen in people of all ages.

Signs and symptoms of heart attack can include one, none, or all of the following:

1. Chest pain or discomfort characterized by a squeezing, crushing, heavy, or burning sensation lasting 2 minutes or more.
2. Pain in the stomach, jaw, neck, left arm, or both arms.
3. Sudden fainting, nausea, or shortness of breath.
4. Unexplained sweating.
5. Pale skin.
6. Anxiety or feeling of impending doom.

Please note, signs and symptoms of heart attack may appear minor and can be easily denied. It is not unusual for a person to make excuses and reject the possibility of heart attack. Research has proven that more than 50 percent of all heart attack victims die outside the hospital, within two hours of the onset of symptoms. When confronted with a possible heart attack patient, *do not* accept excuses; initiate emergency management procedures immediately!

Emergency Management of Heart Attack:

1. Call for an ambulance.
2. Calm and reassure the victim. Explain that help is on the way.
3. Place the victim in a comfortable position, usually sitting because this position eases breathing.
4. *Do not* allow the victim to walk. Movement places further strain on a possibly damaged heart.
5. Be prepared to institute CPR.

Sudden Death

Sudden death may occur from drowning, hypothermia (exposure to cold temperature), severe allergic reactions, injuries to the brain, electrocution, drug overdose, suffocation, severe blood loss, and cardiac arrest due to heart disease. Each of these events may require resuscitative efforts if breathing, or breathing and pulse are absent. *Time is critical!!!!*

The Process of Sudden Death

When breathing and heartbeat stop, a person's bloodstream contains enough reserve oxygen to support life for a few precious minutes. If breathing stops first, the heart will continue to beat until the level of oxygen in the blood becomes too low to support cardiac functioning. Rescue breathing may keep the heart beating.

A person whose heart has stopped beating has an excellent chance of survival if rescue breathing and cardiac compressions (CPR) are started immediately and advanced life support is available as soon as possible to continue care.

The predicament— no breathing or pulse — called *clinical death* is reversible. *Biological death* occurs when brain cells die due to the lack of oxygenated blood; this condition is not reversible.

The goal of CPR is to prevent biological death (brain death). Again, *time is critical.* Minimal brain damage will occur if resuscitative measures are started within 3 to 4 minutes of clinical death.

Types of Sudden Deaths

Drowning

Drowning occurs when a person suffocates in water. At first the drowning victim panics and fights to stay on the surface. Eventually, the air passages and lungs fill with water, or the vocal cords snap shut to prevent water from entering the lungs. In either case, breathing becomes impossible.

Cold water and the *mammalian diving reflex* can extend the time in which a victim, especially a child, can be revived. The mammalian diving reflex is an immediate, natural response to submersion in cold water. It causes the heart rate to slow and blood vessels in the stomach, arms and legs to tighten, which sends oxygenated blood directly to the heart and brain.

Emergency Management of Drowning:

1. Rescue the victim, but be careful not to endanger yourself.
2. Have someone call for an ambulance.
3. Assess breathing. If absent, provide rescue breathing* (See p. 16) Rescue breathing can be started in the water if it is shallow, or on flotation devices if they

allow support of the rescuer and victim.

4. If rescue breathing is ineffective, or if the airway is blocked, use the Heimlich maneuver* to clear the airway.
5. Assess pulse. If pulse is absent, place the victim on a firm surface and start CPR.*
6. Transfer or transport the victim to the hospital for additional care. All victims of drowning or near drowning need physician evaluation.

Hypothermia

Hypothermia is caused by exposure to cold temperatures or by a malfunction of the hypothalmus (the portion of the brain responsible for temperature regulation). In either case, internal body temperature falls to less than 90°F (32° C), and there is a decrease in metabolic activity, pulse rate, and the body's demand for oxygenated blood.

The victim of hypothermia may have slow breathing and pulse rates. If breathing or breathing and pulse are absent, rescue efforts should be initiated and continued until normal body temperature has been restored.

Emergency Management of Hypothermia:

1. Rescue the victim—but only if conditions are safe.
2. Have someone call for an ambulance.
3. Assess breathing and pulse carefully. Pulses may be present but difficult to find. If pulse is absent, start CPR.
4. Cover the victim to prevent further heat loss.
5. Transport the victim to the hospital for additional care and rewarming.

Severe Allergic Reactions

Severe allergic reactions are responses by the body to a specific substance (e.g. insect stings, food, medications, and inhaled matter). Reactions include itching, redness, hives, and swelling in the throat that can develop into upper airway obstruction. People with known allergies should wear medical identification tags.

Special emergency kits are often prescribed for people

*Techniques for rescue breathing, airway obstruction, and cardiac compressions are discussed in detail in the training modules.

with a history of severe allergic reaction. If someone you know carries this kit, learn how to use it.

Emergency Management of Severe Allergic Reactions:

1. Assess breathing and pulse. If absent, start CPR.
2. Have someone call for an ambulance.
3. Transport the victim to the hospital. Special medications will be administered to control signs and symptoms.

Electrocution

Accidental exposure to any electrical source can cause wounds, burns, fractures, and immediate cessation of breathing and pulse. Very often victims of electrical accidents need immediate attention, but these situations call for extreme caution. Exposed wires and energized appliances can electrocute *you.*

Emergency Management of Electrocution:

1. Rescue the victim—but only if conditions are safe and you have proper training and equipment.
2. Have someone call for an ambulance.
3. Assess breathing and pulse. If absent, start CPR.
4. Control severe bleeding at entrance and exit wounds.
5. Transport the victim to the hospital for further care.

Suffocation

People suffocate when something interferes with normal breathing. Causes of suffocation include objects or swelling in the upper airway, gas inhalation, electric shock, drug overdose, and crushing chest injuries. Be especially careful with toxic gases! Some cannot be seen or smelled. Protective breathing apparatus must be worn by trained personnel when rescuing victims of gas inhalation.

Emergency Management of Suffocation:

1. Rescue the victim—but only if conditions are safe!
2. Have someone call for an ambulance.
3. Assess breathing and pulse. If absent, start CPR. Foreign objects in the upper airway can be dislodged by using airway obstruction maneuvers.
4. Transport the victim to the hospital for additional treatment and evaluation.

Trauma

Trauma is an injury produced by a sudden force. Victims of trauma must be handled carefully to avoid causing additional injury. Special care must be taken when any injury to the head or neck is suspected. Avoid twisting the victim's head and neck. Twisting can cause spinal cord damage and even paralysis.

Accidents can cause unsightly injuries. Even though broken bones and open wounds appear life threatening, your attention *must* be directed toward assessing and maintaining breathing and pulse. Profuse bleeding can be controlled by pressing directly on the wound. If necessary, ask someone else to maintain pressure on the wound site while you restore breathing and pulse.

Emergency Management of Trauma:

1. Rescue the victim if life threatening conditions are present. Keep your own safety in mind.
2. Have someone call for an ambulance.
3. Assess breathing and pulse. If absent, start CPR. If turning the victim is necessary, do the following: (Fig. 6)
   - Kneel at the victim's side.
   - Extend the victim's arm—the one nearest you—above his or her head. Straighten or slightly bend the victim's legs at the knees.
   - Support the victim's head and neck with your hand. Reach across the victim's chest and place your other hand under his or her armpit.
   - Roll the victim gently and maintain head support.
   - Turn the victim face up. Avoid twisting the victim's head and neck.
4. Transport the victim to the hospital.

Cardiac Arrest

The most common cause of cardiac arrest in an adult is coronary heart disease; however, any cause of sudden death can lead to cardiac arrest. In infants and children, *respiratory problems* lead to cardiac arrest.

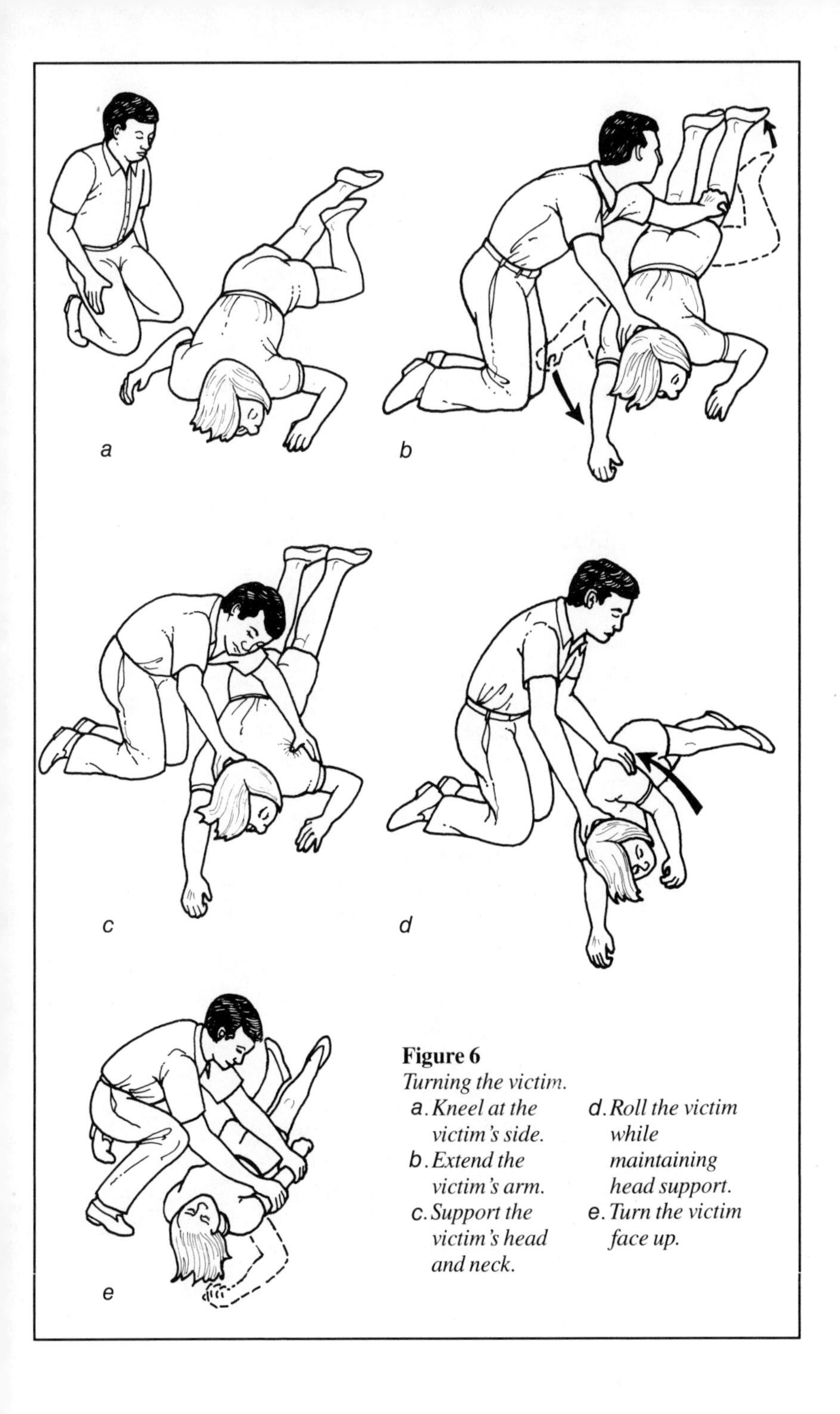

Figure 6
Turning the victim.
a. *Kneel at the victim's side.*
b. *Extend the victim's arm.*
c. *Support the victim's head and neck.*
d. *Roll the victim while maintaining head support.*
e. *Turn the victim face up.*

Cardiac arrest is recognized by the *absence of breathing and pulse.* Recognition and quick action are needed if the victim is to survive. Services provided by ambulance and hospital personnel are only effective when CPR is initiated as soon as possible.

Emergency Management of Cardiac Arrest:

1. Assess breathing and pulse. If absent, start CPR. Have someone call for an ambulance.
2. Transport the victim to the hospital for further treatment.

Certain signs of stroke and seizure may appear similar to cardiac arrest. However, victims of stroke and seizure who have a pulse are *not* in cardiac arrest! Proper assessment is essential for correct treatment.

Stroke

Stroke occurs when a blood vessel in the brain is blocked or bursts. Contributing risk factors include hypertension, heart disease, and diabetes. You should become familiar with the following signs and symptoms of stroke:

1. Sudden loss of consciousness.
2. Paralysis on one or both sides of the body.
3. Facial drooping to one side.
4. Unequal pupils (one larger than the other).
5. Loss of vision in one eye.
6. Severe headache.
7. Speech disturbances (person may be hard to understand or unable to speak).
8. Breathing problems.
9. Nausea, vomiting.
10. Possible convulsions.

The signs and symptoms of stroke may suddenly disappear. This is called a *transient ischemic attack.* Such an occurrence is an early warning sign of stroke. Anyone having any or all of these signs and symptoms should consult a physician for evaluation and treatment.

Emergency Management of Stroke:

1. Assess breathing and pulse. *Check carefully.* If *absent*, start CPR.
2. Have someone call for an ambulance.
3. If breathing and pulse are present:
   a. Calm and reassure the victim.
   b. Do not give the victim anything to drink.
   c. If the victim is conscious, elevate his or her head.
   d. If the victim is unconscious and breathing well, place the person on his or her side with the head tilted backwards and the chin jutting forward. This position provides airway protection. Do not use a pillow.
   e. Cover the victim with a light blanket to maintain body heat.
   f. Do not leave the victim alone.
4. Transport the victim to the hospital for additional care.

Seizures (Convulsions)

Seizures, also called convulsions, can be caused by poisoning, eclampsia (associated with pregnancy), head trauma, diabetic problems, brain tumor, stroke, fever (especially in children), and epilepsy (a disorder characterized by attacks of unconsciousness, with or without muscular contractions). The following are signs and symptoms of seizure:

1. Uncontrolled muscle contractions causing rigidity and jerking followed by a period of relaxation, disorientation, and partial or total unconsciousness.
2. Loss of bowel or bladder control.
3. Temporary blue color to the face.
4. Foaming at the mouth, clenched teeth.
5. Possible sweet breath odor.
6. Lack of breathing during seizure—resumes after seizure.

Seizures can also be nonconvulsive. The person may appear to stare and experience momentary lapse of awareness (absence seizures) or act confused and repeat certain gestures. No prehospital emergency treatment of these seizures is needed; however, the victim should consult a physician for investigation of underlying causes.

Emergency Management of Convulsive Seizures:

During the seizure:

1. Do not restrain the victim.
2. Do not force any object between the victim's teeth.
3. Roll the victim to his or her side, to protect the airway.

After the seizure:

1. Assess breathing and pulse. *Check Carefully!* If *absent,* start CPR.
2. Have someone call an ambulance.
3. If the seizure is a result of trauma, turn the victim carefully (Fig. 6).
4. If breathing and pulse are present:
   a. Reassure the victim.
   b. Do not give the victim anything to eat or drink.
5. If the victim is unconscious but breathing well:
   - Place the victim on his or her side if the seizure was not caused by trauma.
   - Tilt the victim's head backward and jut the chin forward. This position provides airway protection.
   - Do not use a pillow.
6. If the victim is unconscious due to trauma, avoid bending or twisting their neck.
7. Allow the victim to rest.
8. Cover the victim with a light blanket to conserve body heat and prevent embarrassment due to bowel or bladder accident.
9. Transport the victim to the hospital for further care and evaluation.

SECTION 2: CPR FOR ADULTS

Someone needs help! Your heart pounds, your eyes open wide, and your breathing rate increases. Your body is responding to an emergency. Physically you are ready, and after completing CPR training, you will have the knowledge and skills to help. Your emergency plan of action starts with the ABCs.

THE ABCs OF CPR

The ABCs stand for assessment/airway, breathing, and circulation. CPR stands for cardiopulmonary resuscitation (cardio refers to the heart, pulmonary refers to the lungs, and resuscitation means to revive from a condition resembling death).

CPR RATIONALE

The reason CPR is performed is to provide oxygen to the brain, heart, and other organs until medical professionals restore normal breathing and heart action. Speed is critical. Prompt action by trained bystanders saves lives.

CPR SAFETY

Each phase of the ABCs starts with an order for assessment (e.g., determine unresponsiveness, open airway, check breathing, check pulse). Assessment comes first, because rescue techniques that are performed unnecessarily may cause harm. It is important to remember that procedures must *not* be performed until the need has been defined.

The following techniques are to be used on victims over 8 years of age; they should be practiced under the supervision of an instructor. During practice, do not actually perform rescue breathing or cardiac compressions on a classmate or others. These skills are to be performed on a training manikin.

One-Rescuer CPR: Adult
(for Victims over 8 years of Age)

Step 1: Assessment/Airway
Assessment/airway, or the "A" of the ABCs, includes:

- evaluating the scene
- approaching the victim

- determining unresponsiveness: checking for consciousness
- positioning the victim
- opening the airway

Approach the Victim

Use your senses to size up the person's condition as rapidly as possible. Look for signs of movement, signs of breathing, and abnormal position. Was there a fall? Could there be a head or neck injury? If so, move the victim *only if absolutely necessary,* for improper movement can cause paralysis. Look for severe bleeding. If present, have someone press on the wound to control bleeding while you continue with assessment.

Determine Unresponsiveness

Check for consciousness. Is the victim talking to you? If so, have the victim rest quietly and ask someone nearby to call for an ambulance. Do not leave the victim alone. The conscious victim who is struggling to breathe, may have something lodged in the airway. Apply obstructed airway techniques if indicated (see Section 3), and arrange prompt transportation to the hospital.

If the victim does not speak to you, position yourself at their side, tap or gently shake them, keeping in mind the possibility of spinal injury, and ask clearly in a strong voice, "Are you OK?" (Fig. 7). If the victim does not respond, call "Help," and alert others to respond and assist. If you are truly alone, continue rescue procedures (steps 2, 3 and 4) *for 1 minute* before going for help.

Figure 7
Determine unresponsiveness.

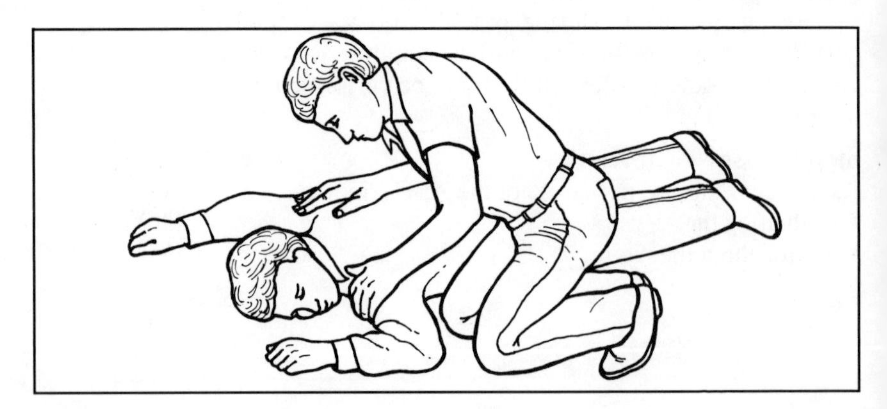

Position the Victim

If CPR is to be effective, the victim must be flat on his or her back, on a firm, flat surface. If the victim is face down, support the head and neck and carefully turn them face up. *Do not* allow the head to roll, twist or tilt backwards or forwards.

Open the Airway

The *tongue* is the most common cause of airway obstruction in the unconscious victim because the relaxed jaw allows the tongue to fall back and close over the airway. The head-tilt/chin-lift maneuver is used to elevate the tongue and open the airway. Follow these steps:

1. Place one hand on the victim's forehead.
2. Apply firm backward pressure.
3. Place index and middle finger of your other hand on the bony part under the edge of the victim's chin.
4. Lift the chin upwards. Avoid closing the mouth. Avoid pressing the flesh under the chin.

Step 2: Breathing

Breathing or the "B" of the ABCs includes:

- checking for signs of breathing
- beginning rescue breathing if the victim is in respiratory arrest

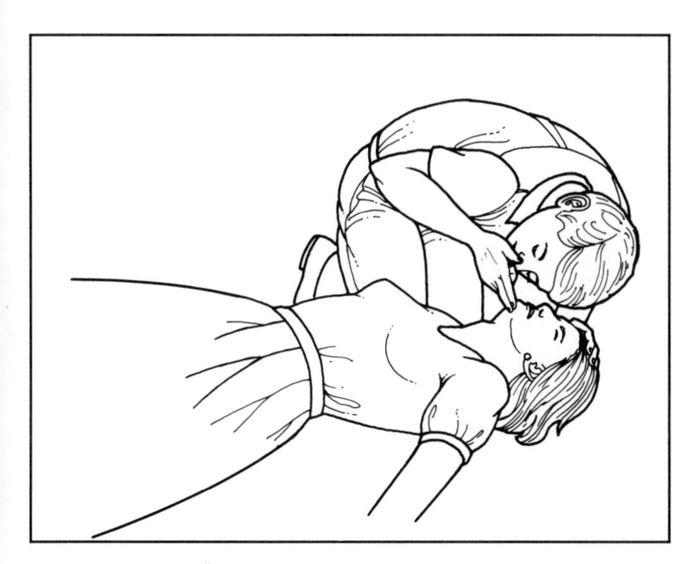

Figure 8
Check breathing.

Check Breathing: Determine Breathlessness

While maintaining an open airway, place your ear close to the victim's mouth and nose for 3 to 5 seconds, and:

- Look: can you see the chest rising?
- Listen: can you hear breathing?
- Feel: can you feel breath on your cheek? (Fig. 8)

If all answers are "Yes," then maintain an open airway and note how often the victim breathes. If all answers are "No," the victim is not breathing and is in respiratory arrest. Rescue breathing is needed.

Provide Rescue Breathing

Provide rescue breathing by mouth-to-mouth, mouth-to-nose, or mouth-to-stoma ventilations. Begin with two ventilations. Your exhaled air contains enough extra oxygen to meet the victim's needs. Follow these steps when providing *mouth-to-mouth* rescue breathing:

1. Maintain head-tilt/chin-lift.
2. Pinch nostrils to prevent air from escaping.
3. Take a deep breath.
4. Seal your mouth over the victim's mouth. Make an airtight seal.

Figure 9
Mouth-to-mouth Rescue Breathing
a. *Maintain head-tilt/chin-lift and pinch the nostrils.*
b. *Seal the mouth and blow slowly.*

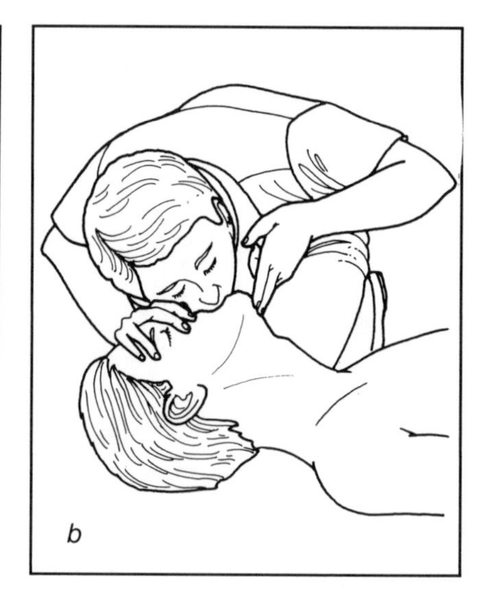

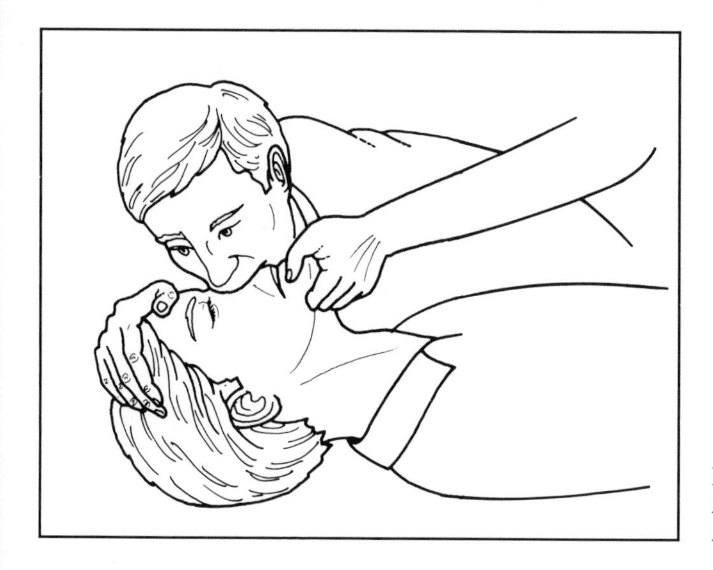

Figure 10
Mouth-to-Nose Rescue Breathing.

5. Blow slowly for 1 to 1.5 seconds, using just enough force to make the chest rise. (Fig. 9)
6. Release the victim's mouth and nose.
7. Allow the victim to exhale.
8. Take a deep breath.
9. Blow slowly again (1 to 1.5 seconds).
10. Allow exhalation.

When injuries, missing teeth, missing dentures, clenched teeth, or other problems make mouth-to-mouth ventilations impossible, use *mouth-to-nose* rescue breathing. Follow these steps:

1. Maintain head-tilt/chin-lift.
2. Lift the victim's jaw and close their mouth with your thumb.
3. Take a deep breath.
4. Seal your mouth over victim's nose.
5. Blow slowly for 1 to 1.5 seconds, using just enough force to make the victim's chest rise. (Fig. 10)
6. Release nose and open the victim's mouth.
7. Allow the victim to exhale.
8. Take a deep breath.
9. Blow slowly again (1 to 1.5 seconds).
10. Release the victim's mouth and nose.
11. Allow exhalation.

Once in a while *mouth-to-stoma* rescue breathing must be provided because the victim has had a laryngectomy which is a surgically created airway connecting the trachea (windpipe) with an opening (stoma) in the base of the person's neck. (Fig. 11) A tracheostomy tube may be in place. Follow these steps:

1. Close the victim's mouth and nose with one hand.
2. Take a deep breath.
3. Seal your mouth over the opening in the neck. Make an airtight seal.
4. Blow slowly through stoma for 1 to 1.5 seconds, using *just* enough force to make the victim's chest rise. (Fig. 12)
5. Release the victim's mouth and nose.
6. Allow the victim to exhale.
7. Take a deep breath.
8. Blow slowly again (1 to 1.5 seconds).
9. Release the victim's mouth and nose.
10. Allow exhalation.

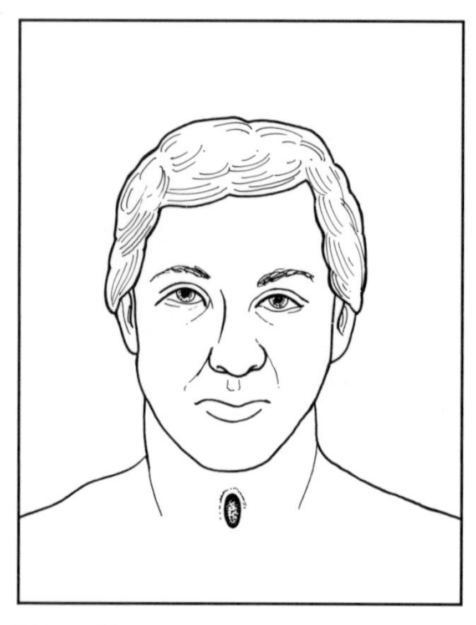

Figure 11
A tracheal stoma.

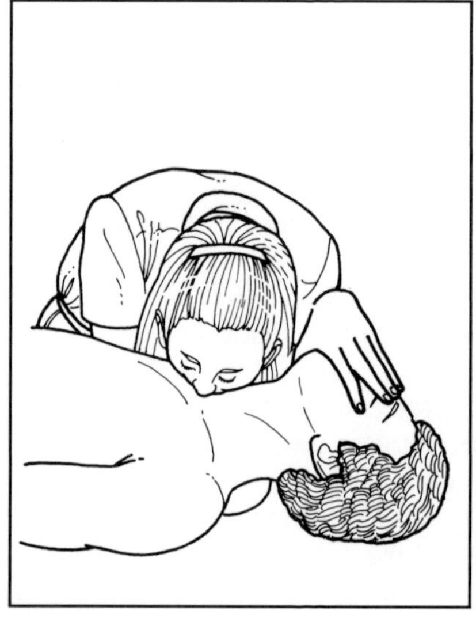

Figure 12
Mouth-to-Stoma Rescue Breathing.

You will know that rescue breathing has been successful when you *see* the victim's chest rise and fall when you *feel* the victim's lungs fill and empty. If rescue breathing attempts are not successful, the tongue may be blocking the airway. Reopen the airway and repeat breaths. If still unsuccessful, a foreign object may have lodged in the airway. Proceed with airway obstruction maneuvers (see Section 3).

Step 3: Circulation

Circulation, or the "C" of the ABCs, includes:

- checking the pulse
- alerting the EMS system
- beginning CPR if the patient is pulseless

Check Pulse: Determining Pulselessness

After providing two full, slow ventilations, check the victim's carotid artery for a pulse. Carotid arteries, which are found in the neck, branch from the aorta and direct blood to the brain. These arteries are considered most reliable because they lie close to the heart, are easily accessible, and will continue to beat after pulses in the arms and wrists are no longer detectable. (Fig. 13) To locate the carotid pulse:

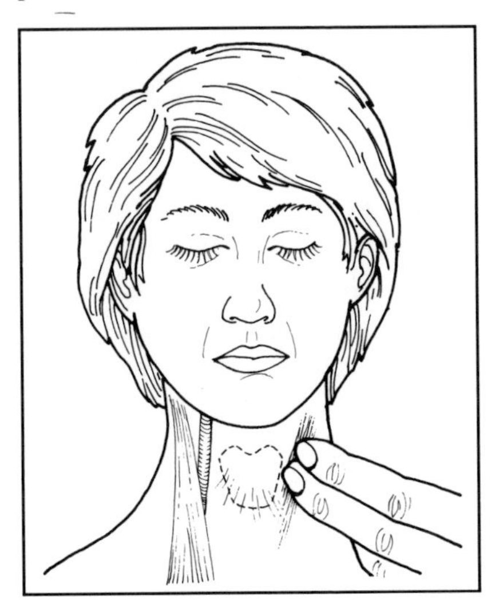

Figure 13
Locate the carotid pulse.

1. Maintain head-tilt with one hand.
2. Touch victim's larynx (Adam's apple) with two or three fingers of your other hand.
3. Slide these fingers toward you into the groove between the trachea and side neck muscles.
4. Press gently for 5 to 10 seconds to check pulsebeat. The pulse may be slow, irregular, very weak and rapid, or absent. Check carefully for this reason: Performing cardiac compressions on a person who has a pulse may disrupt heart rhythm. You can recheck breathing at the same time you are assessing the pulse.

If the pulse is *present,* but the victim isn't breathing, continue rescue ventilations with one breath every 5 seconds (12 times a minute). Count:
1, one thousand,
2, one thousand,
3, one thousand,
4, one thousand,
5, one thousand, breathe.

If the pulse is *absent,* cardiac arrest is confirmed and both rescue breathing *and* cardiac compressions are needed. Make certain the victim is on a *firm* surface. If the victim is in bed, move the person to the floor. If the victim is in a car, move him or her to the ground. A hard surface is needed to perform adequate chest compressions.

Alert EMS System

If someone arrives to help, ask that person to call the emergency telephone number and request an ambulance.

Begin CPR: Begin Chest Compressions

Studies have shown that compressions on the sternum (breast bone) squeeze the heart and increase intrathoracic pressure, creating blood flow. Rescue breathing provides the oxygen, and chest compressions provide the circulation. Chest compressions must *always* be accompanied by rescue breathing.

Proper chest compressions involve locating body landmarks and providing effective downward pressure.

Assume Proper Hand Position

Kneel next to the victim's shoulders. Your upper hand (hand closest to the victim's head) will be maintaining the head-tilt position. Your lower hand (the hand close to the victim's feet) will be lying on their chest. To place both hands properly for CPR, follow these steps:

With your lower hand:

1. locate the lower margin of the victim's rib cage with your index and middle fingers.
2. Run your fingers up the rib cage to the middle of the chest and find the notch at the bottom of the sternum.
3. Place your middle finger in the notch.
4. Place your index finger next to your middle finger.

Figure 14
Proper hand position (adult victim)
a. *Locate the rib margin and sternal notch.*
b. *Place your middle finger in the notch.*

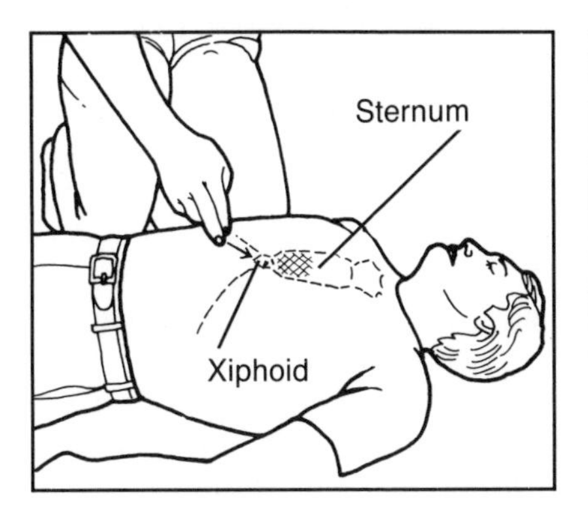

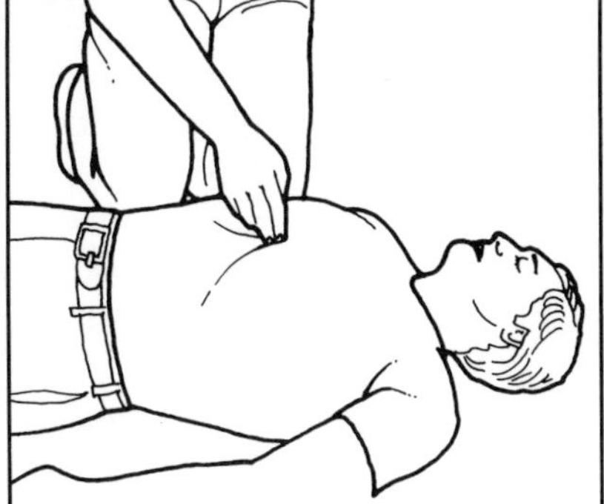

With your upper hand:

5. Release head-tilt.
6. Place the heel of your hand on the long axis of the sternum, next to the fingers of your other hand.
7. Lift your fingers and place your lower hand directly on top of the hand that remains on the sternum. Both hands are parallel.
8. Extend or interlace your fingers. *Do not* allow your fingers to touch the ribs. (Fig. 14)

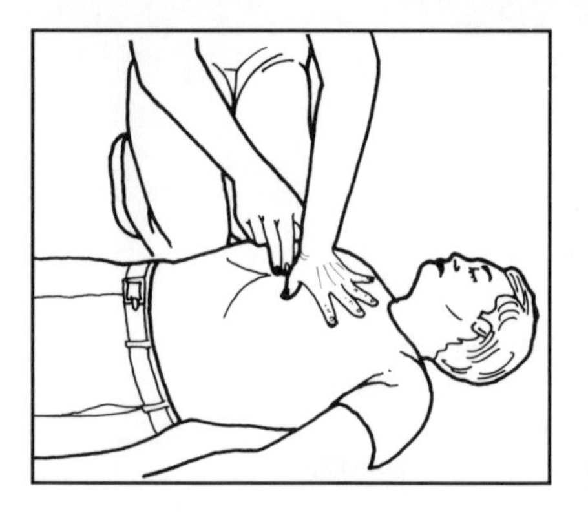

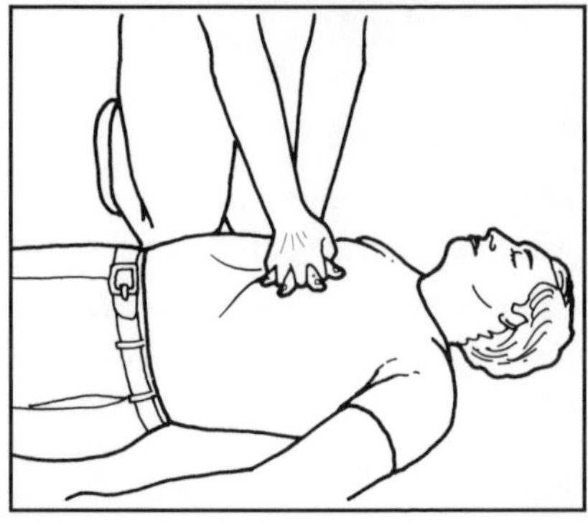

Figure 14 (cont.)
Proper hand position (adult victim)
c. Place your upper hand next to your fingers.
d. Place your lower hand on top of your upper hand.

An alternate method of positioning hands for CPR, which is useful for rescuers who have arthritic hands, is to grasp the wrist of the hand on the chest with the hand that is on the notch at the lower end of the sternum.

Apply Proper Compressions

Now you are ready to begin compressions. Follow these steps:

1. Lock elbows, straighten arms, and position shoulders directly over your hands.
2. Press straight down to depress the sternum 1½ to 2 inches (3.8 to 5.0 cm).
3. Release the chest completely, but *do not* lift your hands from the victim's chest or correct hand position will be lost. (Fig. 15)
4. Deliver smooth and equal (50:50) compressions (downstroke) and relaxation (upstroke) to allow effective blood flow. (Small rescuers may find it easier to deliver compressions by tipping their hips forward on the downstroke and backwards on the upstroke.)
5. Maintain a compression rate of 80 to 100 per minute: count out loud, or to yourself while you press and relax: "One and two and three and four and five and six and seven and eight and nine and ten and eleven and twelve and thirteen and fourteen and fifteen."

Step 4: Compression/Ventilation Cycles

As mentioned earlier, CPR must always be accompanied by rescue breathing. (Fig. 16) To provide proper ventilations, open the airway and deliver two full, slow breaths after 15 compressions. Complete 4 cycles of 15 compressions and 2 ventilations (15:2 ratio).

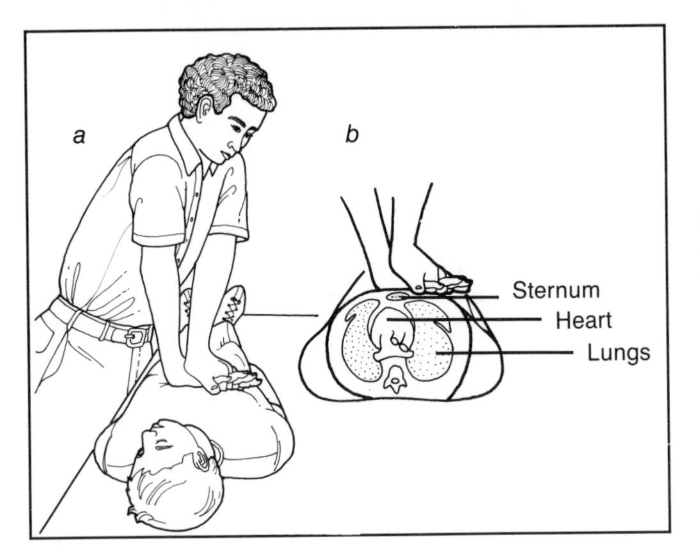

Figure 15
Proper compressions (adult victim)
a. Depress the sternum 1.5 to 2 inches (3.8 to 5.0 cm).
b. Release pressure without lifting your hands.

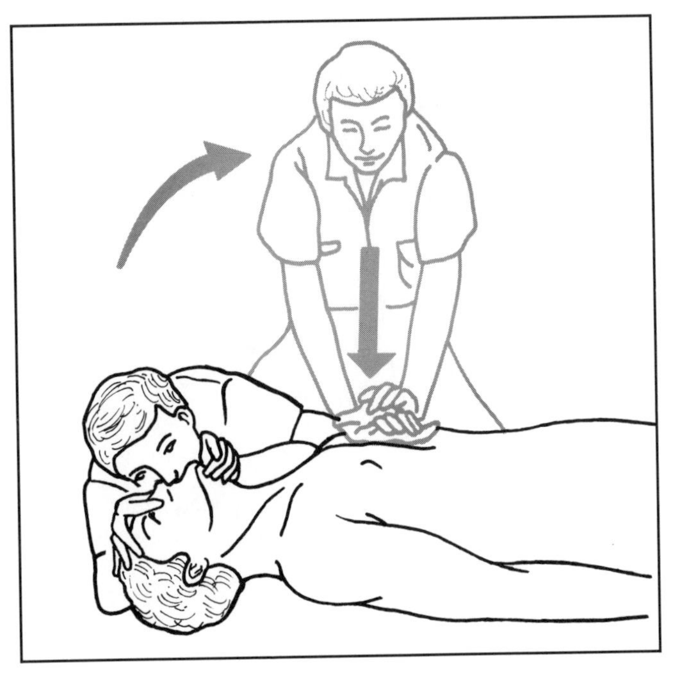

Figure 16
Compressions and ventilations.

Step 5: Reassessment
At the end of 4 compression/ventilation cycles (approximately one minute), reassess breathing and pulse to determine if the patient is recovering. Check breathing and pulse for 5 seconds. If the pulse is *present,* monitor the pulse and breathing. If breathing is *absent,* provide ventilations at the rate of 12 per minute. If the pulse is *absent,* continue CPR. If no one has responded to your cries for help, it is time to leave the victim and call for an ambulance. After contacting the emergency dispatcher, return to the victim and provide further care.

Step 6: Continue CPR
When CPR has to be continued because the patient remains pulseless after reassessment, ventilate two times and resume compressions and ventilations for several minutes. Then check again for the return of breathing and pulse. If absent, continue CPR.

ENTRY OF SECOND RESCUER

Transfer of CPR may take place when another CPR-trained citizen arrives on the scene. The second rescuer should:

1. Announce his or her presence by stating, "I know CPR!"
2. Call the emergency dispatcher and confirm that an ambulance is on the way by announcing, "EMS is activated!"
3. Offer assistance by asking, "Can I help?"

You the first rescuer, decide if help is needed and if a transfer will take place. Follow these steps if you decide to let the second rescuer relieve you.

First Rescuer (you)

1. Complete CPR cycle (15 compressions and 2 ventilations).
2. Say, "Take over CPR!"

Second Rescuer

3. Moves to the victim's head.
4. Opens the airway.

5. Locates the carotid pulse site.
6. Checks pulse and breathing for 5 seconds. If breathing is absent, the second rescuer gives 2 slow, full breaths. If the pulse is absent, the second rescuer starts CPR.

First Rescuer (you)

7. Monitors the victim while the second rescuer performs CPR. The chest should rise during rescue breathing, and a pulse should be felt with each compression. If not, larger breaths and deeper compressions are needed.

Once ambulance personnel arrive, transfer of care occurs after the current rescuer completes a compression/ventilation cycle (15:2).

WHEN TO STOP CPR

Eventually, rescue efforts must cease. You should discontinue CPR when

S—the victim *starts* breathing and has a pulse.
T—you *transfer* care to ambulance personnel or others trained in CPR.
O—you are *out of energy* and can no longer perform CPR.
P—a *physician* is present and assumes responsibility.

CONCERNS/ COMPLICATIONS

Problems with rescue breathing

Vomiting

Vomiting can occur at any time. The unconscious victim must be handled carefully, because vomitus in the lungs (aspiration) is life-threatening. Aspiration may cause a type of pneumonia that can kill the victim even after rescue efforts have been successful.

At the first sign of vomiting:

1. Turn the victim to the side.
2. Maintain this position until vomiting ends.
3. Wipe vomit out of the victim's mouth. Use your fingers or a cloth.
4. Reposition the victim on his or her back if rescue breathing is needed.
5. Resume rescue breathing if indicated.

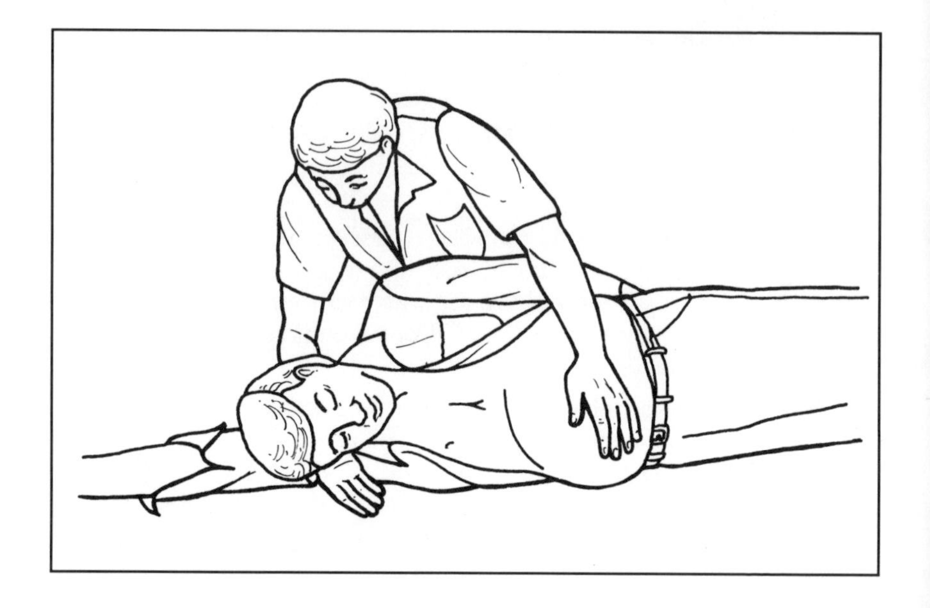

Figure 17
Severe gastric distension. If distension interferes with rescue breathing, turn the victim to the side, press upper abdomen and expect vomiting.

Gastric Distension

Gastric distension (air in the stomach) occurs when rescue breathing is performed too quickly or too forcefully, or when the victim's airway is partially or completely blocked. Too much air in the stomach can cause vomiting and may limit lung expansion.

At the first sign of gastric distension:

1. Reopen victim's airway.
2. Slow rescue breathing to 1 to 1.5 seconds per inflation.
3. Reduce ventilations. Blow just enough to make the victim's chest rise.

If *severe* gastric distension elevates the diaphragm, limits lung expansion, and interferes with rescue breathing:

1. Turn the victim to the side.
2. Press their upper abdomen. *Do not* maintain continuous pressure because you may damage the liver. (Fig. 17)

3. Expect vomiting. When the victim has finished vomiting wipe any vomit out of their mouth.
4. Reposition the victim on his or her back.
5. Resume rescue breathing if needed.

Loose or Broken Teeth, Dentures, or Dental Appliances
Loose or broken teeth, dentures, or dental appliances must be removed to avoid creating an upper airway obstruction and/or blowing fragments into the victim's lungs. Secure dentures should be left in place because rescue breathing techniques are much easier when dentures remain in the victim's mouth.

The unresponsive, nonbreathing and pulseless victim *must* receive a combination of rescue breathing and external chest compressions in order to survive cardiac arrest. Even though compressions will cause rib fractures and internal injuries in some victims, these injuries can be repaired after resuscitation.
To minimize injuries and provide adequate compressions:

1. Find proper landmarks and *avoid* pressing over the tip of the sternum (xiphoid process).
2. Interlock or elevate fingers and *avoid* pressing on ribs.
3. Evaluate depth of compression: 1.5 to 2 inches (3.8 to 5 cm) is needed to create blood flow. Shallow compressions may be ineffective, and deeper compressions may cause injury.
4. Evaluate the type of compression: Smooth, even strokes are needed to allow heart filling. Jerky, stabbing compressions decrease blood flow.

   CPR must be started as soon as safely possible; however, movement of the victim from the scene must wait until ambulance personnel arrive and moving CPR can be performed without interruption.

SECTION 3: UPPER AIRWAY OBSTRUCTION IN ADULTS

More people die from upper airway obstruction caused by unconsciousness than by foreign body obstruction. If attempts to open the airway using the head-tilt/chin-lift maneuver and to provide rescue breathing (twice) prove unsuccessful in the unconscious victim, then it must be assumed a foreign object is blocking the airway.

In 1981, 3,100 people died because foreign objects such as food or small items caught in their upper airway. The term "cafe coronary" has been used to describe a choking incident in a restaurant, when upper airway obstruction has been mistaken for heart attack.

Foreign body obstruction can be avoided if people will:

- Cut food into small, easily chewed pieces.
- Limit alcohol intake.
- Avoid laughing and talking while eating.
- Make certain dentures fit snugly.
- Keep small objects away from infants and small children.
- Not allow children to walk or run with food in their mouths.

RECOGNIZING FOREIGN BODY OBSTRUCTION

Objects in the upper airway may allow some airflow. Management of partial airway obstruction depends on the victim's breathing efforts. Check their breathing. Is the victim displaying good or poor air exchange? With good air exchange, the victim will cough forcefully and may wheeze between coughs. With poor air exchange, the victim:

- Will cough weakly.
- Will strain to breathe.
- May make high-pitched, crowing sounds.
- May show blueness of the lips and fingernails (cyanosis).

A complete airway obstruction blocks all airflow. Recognition of complete airway obstruction depends on the victim's state of consciousness. The *conscious* victim cannot cough, breath, or speak, and may stagger about, neck straining, while clutching his or her throat (the *universal distress signal*). (Fig. 18)

The *unconscious* victim may have visible signs of upper airway obstruction—the rescuer can see the object(s), or the obstruction may not be discovered until rescue breathing attempts are made—the rescuer will be unable to ventilate the victim.

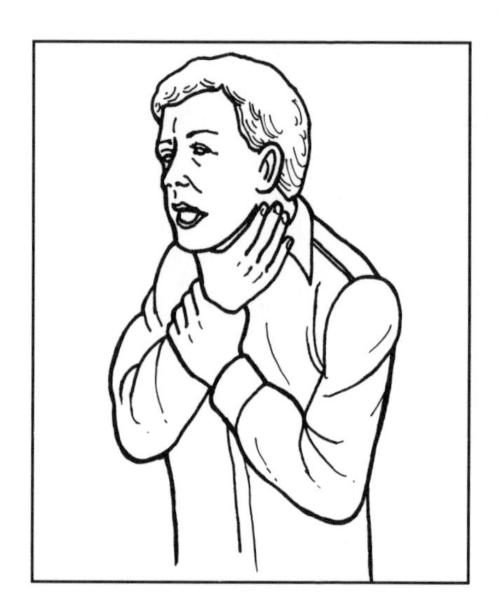

Figure 18
The universal distress signal indicating choking.

MANAGEMENT OF OBSTRUCTED AIRWAY IN A CONSCIOUS ADULT

The following techniques are used on victims over eight years of age. They are to be practiced under the supervision of your instructor. During practice, do not actually perform the Heimlich maneuver, jaw-tongue lift, finger sweeps, or rescue breathing on a classmate. Some of these skills may be performed on a training manikin.

Step 1: Assessment/Airway
Evaluate the scene. Make sure conditions are safe for yourself and the person in need.

Approach the victim. Is the person staggering, neck straining, eyes open wide, and hands grasping their throat? This is the *universal distress signal* indicating choking.

Ask the person, "Are you choking?" If the victim speaks and coughs forcefully, this indicates *good air exchange.* Encourage the person to cough. Coughing is nature's way of clearing upper airway obstruction. Do avoid slapping the person on their back. Stay with the victim and be prepared to help if signs of poor air exchange develop. If partial obstruction persists, call for an ambulance.

With poor exchange, locate appropriate landmarks and perform the Heimlich maneuver.

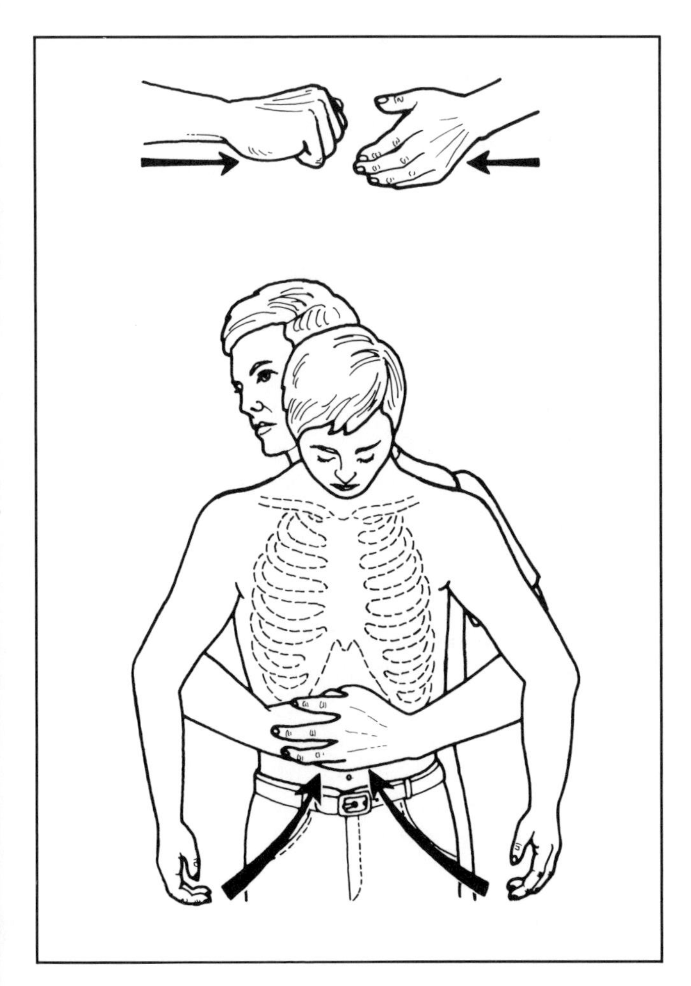

Figure 19 *Performing abdominal thrusts (Heimlich Maneuver) on a standing or seated victim.*

Step 2: Heimlich Maneuver

The Heimlich maneuver, invented by Dr. Henry Heimlich, consists of abdominal thrusts which force air out of the lungs and propel the obstruction up the airway. This technique can be performed while the victim is standing, sitting, or lying.

Abdominal Thrusts (Heimlich Maneuver)

When the victim is standing or sitting, perform the Heimlich maneuver following these steps:

1. Stand directly behind the victim.
2. Wrap your arms around the victim's waist. Keep your elbows out, away from the victim's ribs.
3. Make a fist with one hand. Place thumb side of your fist on the victim's upper abdomen, just above their navel, and well below the tip of the sternum (xiphoid process).
4. Grasp your fist with your other hand.
5. Provide swift, inward and upward thrusts until the object is released or victim becomes unconscious. (Fig. 19)

Chest Thrusts

An alternate Method for Obese or Pregnant Victims

If a victim is extremely obese, encircling the waist may be impossible, or if the victim is in her last months of pregnancy, there may not be room between the enlarged uterus and the rib cage to perform abdominal thrusts. In both cases chest thrusts should be used instead of abdominal thrusts. Follow these steps:

1. Stand directly behind the victim.
2. Wrap your arms around the victims's chest, under the victim's armpits.
3. Keep your arms away from the victim's ribs.
4. Make a fist with one hand. Place thumb side on middle of the victim's sternum. *Do not press on ribs or lower end of sternum* (xiphoid process).

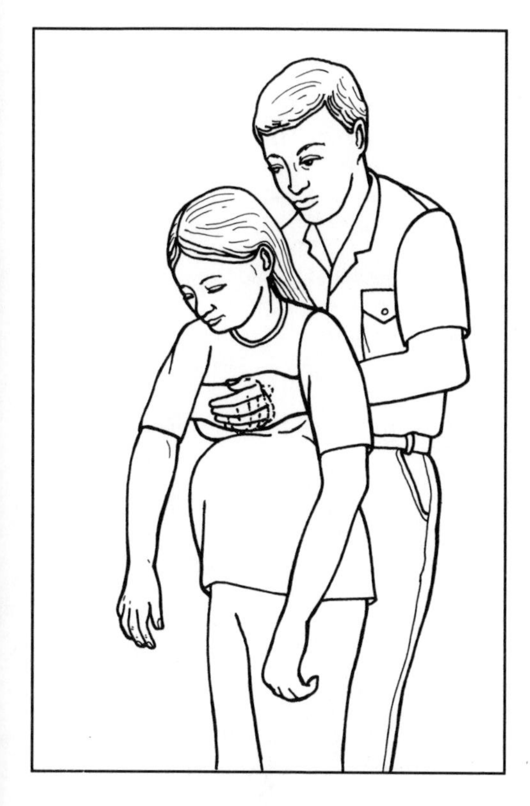

Figure 20
Performing chest thrusts on a pregnant patient.

5. Grasp your fist with your other hand.
6. Provide swift *backward* thrusts, until the object is released or the victim becomes unconscious. (Fig. 20)

If You are Alone and Choking

Probably everyone has at some time or another experienced the fear of choking. Usually, a good, hard cough does the trick. But what if you had a serious problem and no one was around to assist you? Then help yourself! Learn this simple procedure:

1. Make a fist with one hand.

2. Place the thumb side of your fist just above your navel.
3. Grasp the fist with your other hand.
4. Press inward and upward until the object is released.
5. If unsuccessful, lean over a firm object (chairback, table, etc.) and press quickly. (Fig. 21)

If Victim Is Lying Down

If the victim has fallen, but is still conscious:

1. Position the victim face upward.
2. Keep the victim's chin in line with the sternum. This allows proper movement of the object up the airway.
3. Straddle the victim's thighs.
4. Place the heel of one hand in the mid-abdominal area, above the navel and well below the tip of the sternum (xiphoid process).

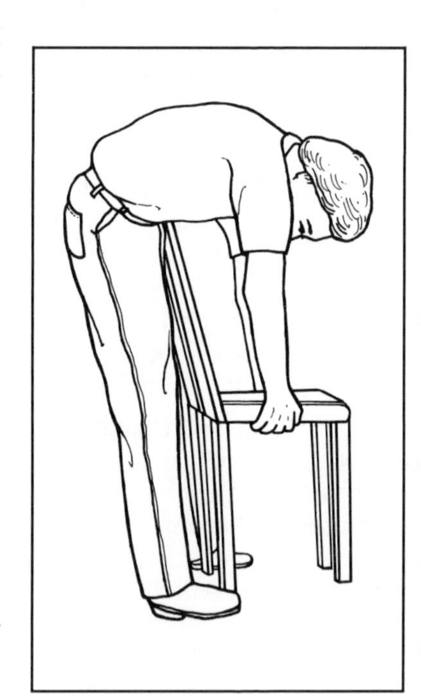

Figure 21
Self help for upper airway obstruction.

5. Place your other hand on top of the first hand. You may interlock fingers.
6. Provide swift inward and upward thrusts until the object is released or the victim becomes unconscious. (Fig.22)

If the victim is extremely obese or pregnant, position him or her face upward, chin in line with sternum. Find landmarks for performing cardiac compressions and provide downward chest thrusts until the object is released, or the victim becomes unconscious.

If at any time the *victim starts coughing, stop and evaluate air exchange.* With good air exchange, monitor breathing and arrange transportation to the hospital. With poor air exchange, continue rescue procedures.

Step 3: Additional Assessment (For the Victim Who Becomes Unconscious)

Lack of oxygen will cause unconsciousness. *Be alert!* The victim can become unconscious at any time. The rescuer must be prepared to assist the victim who becomes unconscious.

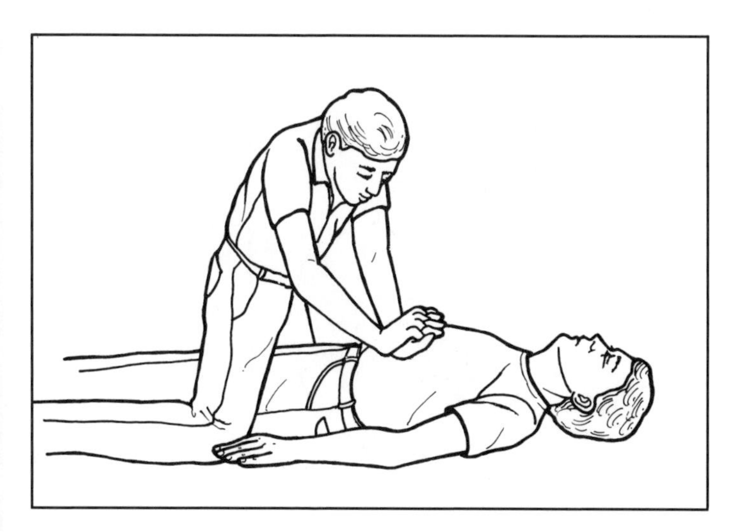

Figure 22 *Performing abdominal thrusts (Heimlich Maneuver) astride.*

Position the Victim

Do not allow the victim to fall. Brace yourself and lower the victim to the floor. Place the victim face up, chin in line with the sternum. Do not twist the neck.

Call For Help

Shout, "Help!" If someone responds, direct the person to call the emergency number and request an ambulance.

Step 4: Foreign Body Check (For Unconscious Victims Only)

Open the victim's airway with the tongue-jaw lifting maneuver (Fig. 23). Grasp the victim's tongue and lower jaw between your thumb and fingers. Lift the jaw upward. If you are unable to open the victim's mouth, use the cross-finger technique:

1. Place your thumb on the victim's lower teeth.
2. Place your index finger on victim's upper teeth.
3. Push the teeth apart.
4. Perform finger sweep.

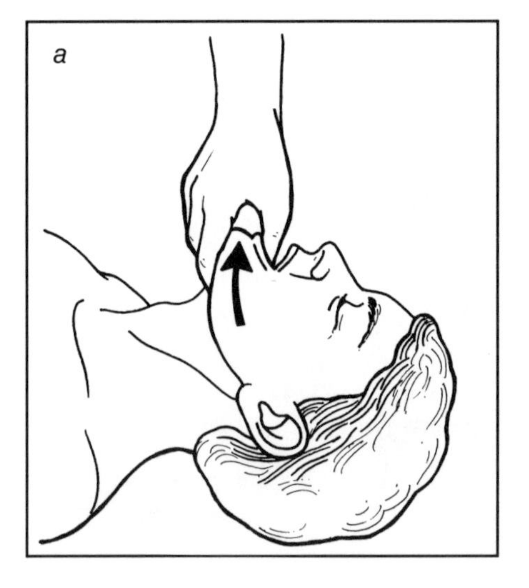

Figure 23
Foreign body check and finger sweep.
a. *Use the tongue-jaw lift to open the airway.*

Look for the foreign object. If you see it, remove it with the thumb and index finger of your available hand, then check breathing and pulse.

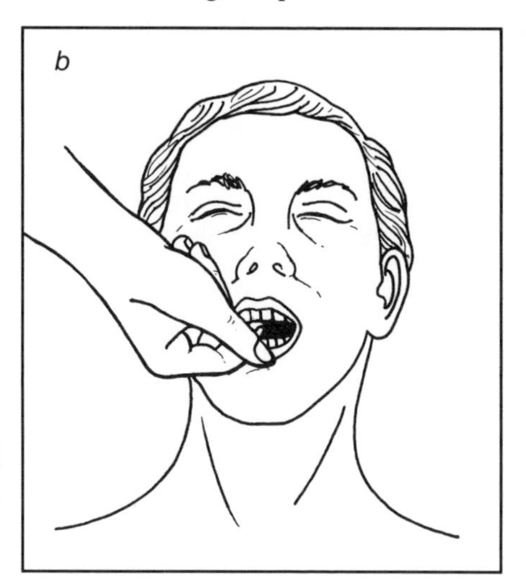

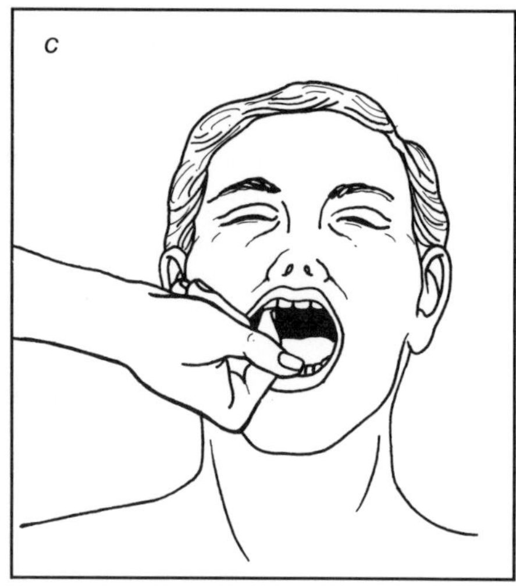

Figure 23 (cont.)
b. & c. *If the mouth is closed, use the cross-finger technique.*
d. *Perform a finger sweep and attempt to remove the obstruction.*

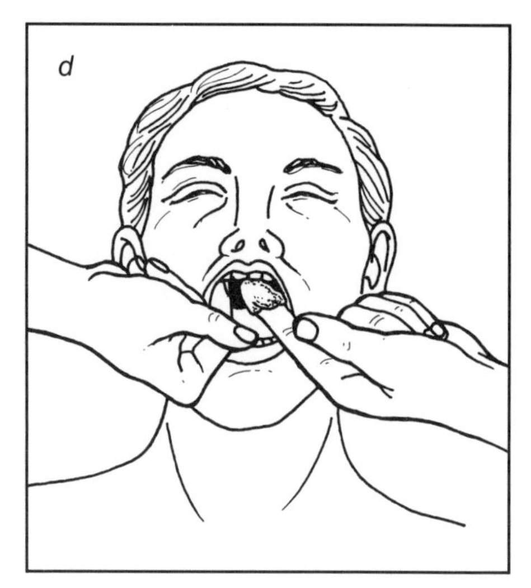

If the object is not in sight, perform a finger sweep using this technique:

1. Maintain open airway with one hand.
2. Hook the index finger of your other hand and sweep the throat. Take care! Do not push the object deeper into the airway. (Fig. 23)
3. If the object is loosened, grasp and remove it. Evaluate breathing and pulse.
4. If the object is not loosened, try rescue breathing. Forceful breaths may bypass the obstruction.

Step 5: Ventilation

Having completed a foreign body check, try ventilating the unconscious victim. Open the airway using the head-tilt/chin-lift maneuver. Attempt ventilations using mouth-to-mouth or mouth-to-nose techniques. If successful, provide two rescue breaths and check pulse. If ventilations are *not* successful, perform the Heimlich maneuver.

Step 6: Heimlich Maneuver

Position the victim face upward, chin in line with sternum. Straddle victim's thighs and provide 6 to 10 swift inward and upward abdominal thrusts.

Step 7: Foreign Body Check

Open the airway. Grasp the victim's jaw and tongue and lift upward. Perform a finger sweep, sweeping deeply from one cheek to the other. If the object still cannot be removed, try rescue breathing.

Step 8: Rescue Breathing Attempt

Attempt ventilating again. If successful, provide two rescue breaths and check the carotid pulse.

Step 9: Sequencing

If after completing Steps 1 to 8 you have not been able to revive the victim, begin sequencing—that is, repeat the Heimlich maneuver, finger sweeps, and ventilations (steps 6 to 8) until the object is released and/or ambulance personnel take over care of the victim. Keep in mind that a lack of oxygen will cause muscles to relax. Rescue procedures may loosen the object, or allow ventilations to bypass the obstruction. Keep trying!

MANAGEMENT OF OBSTRUCTED AIRWAY IN AN UNCONSCIOUS ADULT

When approaching a victim who appears to be unconscious, the rescuer may not realize the problem is foreign body obstruction until rescue breathing has been attempted and is unsuccessful.

Step 1: Assessment/Airway

1. *Evaluate the scene.* Make sure conditions are safe for you and the person in need. Approach the victim. Use your senses to rapidly size up his or her condition.
2. *Determine unresponsiveness.* If the victim appears unconscious, position yourself at the victim's side, tap or gently shake the person's shoulders, keeping in mind possible spinal injury, and ask in a firm voice, "Are you OK?" If the victim remains unresponsive, you may have to turn him. You must also call for help. Shout "Help!" and alert others to respond and assist.
3. *Position the victim.* If necessary, turn the victim on his or her back while supporting the head and neck.
4. *Open the airway.* Remember, the tongue is the most common cause of airway obstruction in the unconscious victim. Perform the head-tilt/chin-lift maneuver to open the airway.
5. *Check breathing: determine breathlessness.* While maintaining an open airway, look, listen and feel for breathing efforts for 3 to 5 seconds. If the victim is breathing, maintain an open airway and monitor by looking, listening, and feeling. If the victim is not breathing or shows signs of poor air exchange, attempt rescue breathing.

Step 2: Breathing Attempt

1. *Attempt ventilation.* While maintaining an open airway, provide rescue ventilations using the mouth-to-mouth or mouth-to-nose techniques. If successful, provide two rescue breaths and check the carotid

pulse. If *not* successful, the airway is blocked. Reopen the airway and ventilate again.

2. *Reattempt ventilations.* Reposition the victim's head to open the airway. Seal the mouth and nose. Provide rescue ventilations. If not successful, activate EMS and perform the Heimlich maneuver.
3. *Activate EMS system.* Direct someone to call the emergency dispatcher and request an ambulance.

Step 3: Heimlich Maneuver

Perform abdominal thrusts while waiting for the ambulance:

1. Position the victim face upward, chin in line with sternum.
2. Straddle the victim's thighs.
3. Provide 6 to 10 swift, inward and upward thrusts. For obese or pregnant victims, find landmarks for performing cardiac compressions and provide 6 to 10 downward thrusts.

Step 4: Foreign Body Check

After performing 6 to 10 thrusts, perform a finger sweep:

1. Open the airway.
2. Grasp the jaw and tongue. Lift upward.
3. Provide finger sweep with index finger. Sweep deeply, from one cheek to the other.

Step 5: Breathing Attempt

Attempt to ventilate the victim. If successful, provide two rescue breaths and check the carotid pulse. If *not* successful, repeat procedures.

Step 6: Sequencing

Repeat the Heimlich maneuver, finger sweep, and ventilations (steps 3 to 5) until the object is released and/or ambulance personnel take over care of the victim. If the unconscious victim starts coughing, *stop* and evaluate air exchange. With *good air exchange*, position the victim on his or her side, monitor breathing, and make sure the patient is transported to the hospital. With *poor air exchange,* repeat all the procedures.

CONCERNS AND COMPLICATIONS

All victims of airway obstruction must be evaluated by a physician because:

1. Foreign objects may cause bleeding and swelling.
2. The Heimlich maneuver may cause internal injuries.
3. Small objects may drop or be blown into the lungs.

To minimize injuries/complications:

1. Assess the victim and follow correct procedures.
2. Find proper landmarks and *avoid* pressing on ribs or the tip of the sternum (xiphoid process).
3. Arrange transportation of the victim to the hospital for additional care and evaluation.

ADULT MODULE: QUESTIONS/ANSWERS

The following questions are based on the information found in sections 2 and 3. Circle the letter of the correct answer.

1. The ABCs stand for:
   a. Approach, Breathe, and Circulate.
   b. Assessment/Airway, Breathing, and Circulation.
   c. Assessment/Airway, Breathing, and Compression.
   d. Approach, Beware, and Circumvent.
2. CPR stands for:
   a. cardiovascular pulmonary resection.
   b. common sense revelation.
   c. cardiac patient research.
   d. cardiopulmonary resuscitation.
3. State of consciousness can be determined by:
   a. slapping the victim's face and pinching shoulder muscles.
   b. tickling the soles of the victim's feet.
   c. Asking, "Are you OK?" and gently shaking the victim.
   d. whispering in the victim's ear.
4. Vomit is the most common cause of airway obstruction in the unconscious victim.
   a. true
   b. false
5. To check breathing, open the airway and
   a. place the palm of your hand over the victim's mouth and nose.
   b. use a mirror and check for fogging.
   c. place your ear close to the victim's mouth and nose and look for chest rise and fall.
   d. place your ear on the victim's chest and listen for breath sounds.
6. When providing mouth-to-nose rescue breathing, lift the jaw, close the victim's mouth, and blow through the victim's nostrils.
   a. true
   b. false

7. The carotid pulse is located in the
   a. hip.
   b. arm.
   c. neck.
   d. ankle.
8. The carotid pulse is considered most reliable because
   a. it is easily accessible.
   b. it lies close to the heart.
   c. it will continue to beat after other pulses are no longer detectable.
   d. all of the above.
9. If the unresponsive victim's pulse is present,
   a. monitor pulse and provide rescue breathing if needed.
   b. immediately leave the victim and contact the emergency dispatcher.
   c. give the patient sips of water.
   d. all of the above.
10. Adequate cardiac compressions can be performed on the victim who is
    a. seated in a chair.
    b. floating in the water.
    c. lying on the floor.
    d. lying on a bed.
11. To find compression landmarks
    a. locate the victim's trachea (windpipe) and run your fingers down the neck until you reach the top of the sternum.
    b. locate bottom of the victim's rib cage, run your fingers up the ribs to the middle of the chest, and place your middle finger in the notch at the lower end of the sternum.
    c. locate nipple line and place the heel of one hand crosswise on the victim's sternum.
    d. locate nipple line and place the heel of both hands lengthwise on the long axis of the victim's sternum.
12. When performing cardiac compressions,
    a. position your shoulders directly over the sternum.
    b. depress sternum 1.5 to 2 inches (3.8 to 5.0 cm).

c. release chest on upstroke without lifting hands off the sternum.
d. all of above.

13. To minimize rib fractures
    a. locate compression landmarks.
    b. keep hands and/or fingers off ribs.
    c. judge proper compression depth.
    d. all of the above.
14. The ratio of compressions to ventilations in adult: one-rescuer CPR is:
    a. 2:15
    b. 15:2
    c. 60:2
    d. 5:3
15. Pulse checks should take place after initial ventilations, after the first minute of CPR, and every few minutes thereafter.
    a. true
    b. false
16. It is all right to stop CPR when you are exhausted.
    a. true
    b. false
17. If vomiting occurs,
    a. continue rescue breathing as victim vomits.
    b. immediately discontinue rescue procedures because vomiting means the victim cannot be resuscitated.
    c. stop, turn the victim to the side, and wait until vomiting finishes.
    d. stop rescue breathing and begin chest compressions.
18. Gastric distention is a result of
    a. foreign body obstruction.
    b. inadequate head-tilt/chin-lift.
    c. overventilating.
    d. all of the above.
19. Mouth-to-mouth rescue breathing is much easier if the victim's dentures are left in place.
    a. true
    b. false

20. If the pulse is present, but the adult victim isn't breathing,
    a. provide 1 rescue breath every 6 seconds.
    b. provide 2 rescue breaths every 2 seconds.
    c. provide 1 rescue breath every 5 seconds.
    d. provide 2 rescue breaths every 4 seconds.
21. Loose dentures may lead to upper airway obstruction.
    a. true
    b. false
22. Use of the head-tilt/chin-lift may relieve upper airway obstruction.
    a. true
    b. false
23. Partial airway obstruction may allow some air to bypass the object.
    a. true
    b. false
24. Signs of upper airway obstruction include
    a. coughing (weak or forceful).
    b. high-pitched, crowing sounds.
    c. cyanosis.
    d. all of the above.
25. With complete airway obstruction,
    a. the victim will cough forcefully and wheeze between coughs.
    b. the victim will be unable to cough, breathe, or speak.
    c. the rescuer may not discover the obstruction until attempting to ventilate the victim.
    d. both b and c are correct.
26. It is impossible to perform the Heimlich maneuver on yourself.
    a. true
    b. false
27. When performing the Heimlich maneuver on the conscious, standing victim,
    a. position yourself at the victim's side, hug the victim's ribs, and press inward.
    b. position yourself behind the victim, place your fist above the victim's waist, and administer thrusts.

c. stand in front of the victim, place the heel of your hand on the victim's chest, and push rapidly.
d. stand in front of the victim, place the heel of your hand on the victim's upper abdomen, and push rapidly.

28. When performing the Heimlich Maneuver, special care should be take to avoid pressing on the
    a. femur and patella.
    b. humerus and tibia.
    c. ribs and xiphoid process.
    d. radius and ulna.
29. When performing the Heimlich maneuver on the victim who is lying down, turn the victim's head to the side for better airway management.
    a. true
    b. false
30. In the unconscious victim, the foreign body check can be performed using the tongue-jaw lift or cross-finger technique.
    a. true
    b. false
31. The finger sweep may loosen the object enough to allow rescue breathing to bypass the obstruction.
    a. true
    b. false
32. All victims of airway obstruction must be evaluated by a physician because
    a. the victim's airway may swell after the obstruction is removed.
    b. rescue techniques may cause injuries.
    c. small objects may have dropped into the lungs.
    d. all of the above.

ANSWERS

1.–b	9.–a	17.–c	25.–d
2.–d	10.–c	18.–d	26.–b
3.–c	11.–b	19.–a	27.–b
4.–b	12.–d	20.–c	28.–c
5.–c	13.–d	21.–a	29.–b
6.–a	14.–b	22.–a	30.–a
7.–c	15.–a	23.–a	31.–a
8.–d	16.–a	24.–d	32.–d

SECTION 4: CPR FOR INFANTS AND CHILDREN

You've heard the warnings: "Lock up medicines!" "Don't play with matches!" "Plastic bags suffocate!" "Mr. Yuk means poison!" "Buckle Up!" These warnings have special meaning when you realize accidents are the leading cause of death in infants and children. According to the National Center of Health Statistics, nearly 9,000 pediatric deaths occur annually. According to the American Academy of Pediatrics, four times as many children die from car accidents, choking, suffocation, poisoning, burns and electrocution as from any childhood disease. Tragically, most accidents are preventable.

ACCIDENTS THAT SHOULD NOT HAPPEN

Motor Vehicle Accidents

Statistics show most children over the age of 1 year die as a result of traffic accidents. The primary reason is failure to use proper restraints. Small children *must* be buckled into crash-tested automobile safety seats. Large children *and* adults must buckle seat belts. In 1981, nearly 50,000 people died from automobile injuries. In countries where seat belts are mandatory, automobile fatalities have decreased by as much as 40 percent.

Airway Obstruction/Suffocation/Strangulation

Infants and small children explore with their mouths, and objects can lodge in the airway limiting breathing. The following suggestions will help prevent airway problems:

1. Do not allow small toys, balloons, and toys with detachable parts.
2. Remove button eyes and noses from stuffed animals.
3. Survey your home and remove small objects (e.g., buttons, pins marbles, coins, nuts) from baby's environment.
4. Hold your baby while bottle feeding. Propped bottles may cause choking.
5. Choose snacks appropriate for the age of child. Popcorn and nuts, for example, should not be given to young children.
6. Do not allow children to walk or run with food or other items in their mouths.

7. Set a good example—keep safety pins out of *your* mouth.
8. Remember, thin plastic causes suffocation. When disposing of plastic bags, first tie them in knots. *Do not* cover crib mattress with thin plastic film.
9. Take doors and lids off empty trunks and appliances.
10. Think safety when selecting a crib. Make sure the slats are no more than 2 3/8 inches apart to prevent the baby from slipping through. The mattress should fit tightly to ends and sides.
11. *Nothing* should be hung around baby's neck, including pacifiers, rattles, necklaces, or religious objects.
12. Toys hung across the crib should be removed before baby can sit up.
13. Toys hung from the side of the crib should be short—less than 5 inches long.
14. Be careful with cords (e.g., electrical, drapery, telephone) that can cause objects to fall and may strangulate.

Poisoning

The world is full of attractively packaged, fragrant, and sweet-tasting products that are designed to make our lives easier. Unfortunately, many of these products are poisonous. A curious child cannot read or may ignore warning statements, so adults must be aware of dangerous substances. The following suggestions will help prevent accidental poisoning:

1. Store all medicines out of children's reach.
2. Do not describe a child's medicine as "candy."
3. Consider all manufactured products poisonous. Poisonous products include detergents, waxes, drain cleaners, fuel oil, paint thinner, mothballs, weed killer, fertilizer, pesticides, hair spray, nail polish, and eye makeup.
4. Keep all products in their original containers.,
5. Suspect all plants, including house plants. Some are extremely toxic.
6. Keep alcoholic beverages and products (e.g., mouthwash, cough syrup) out of children's reach.

7. Choose nontoxic, lead-free finishes when renovating toys or furniture.
8. Teach children to ask permission before touching, tasting, or smelling unfamiliar items.
9. Keep syrup of ipecac handy, but contact poison control or a physician *before* giving any treatment for poisoning.

Fires/Electric Shock/Other Accidents

Burns, electrocution, drowning, and falls cause injuries and death. The following suggestions promote a safe environment:

1. Store matches, lighters, and flammable liquids safely.
2. Place smoke detectors with fresh batteries on all levels of your home.
3. Hold periodic fire drills. Plan escape routes and a rendezvous place away from the home. Stress keeping low to avoid breathing noxious fumes.
4. Buy flame-retardant clothing. By law, all clothing up to 6X is flame-retardant.
5. Place "Totfinder" stickers on children's bedroom windows and on the door, 2 inches from the floor.
6. Keep appliance cords out of children's reach.
7. Unplug and store unused cords.
8. Cover or tape with electrical tape unused outlets.
9. Teach children to swim.
10. Supervise children while swimming or bathing.
11. Set tap water at 120 degrees Farenheit to avoid scalding.
12. Avoid drinking hot beverages while holding a child.
13. Turn pot handles away from the front of the stove.
14. Screen fireplaces, radiators, heaters, and coal and wood-burning stoves to prevent burning.
15. Prevent falls by
    - keeping stairways clear.
    - barricading stairways with safety gates.
    - positioning crib mattress low, and crib sides high.
    - never leaving baby unattended on a bed or on a changing table.
    - lifting and belting children into highchairs and walkers. Do not allow the child to climb.
    - screening and locking low windows.
    - skidproofing rugs and tubs.

Motor vehicle accidents, airway obstruction, suffocation, strangulation, poisoning, fires, electrical shock, accidental falls can cause sudden death in adults and children alike. However, unlike adults, very few children die from cardiac problems. *Respiratory (breathing) problems* are the main cause of cardiac arrest in infants and small children.

An emergency plan of action for the infant or child in need starts with the ABCs.

THE ABCs OF CPR

The ABCs stand for assessment/airway, breathing and circulation. CPR stands for cardiopulmonary resuscitation: cardio refers to the heart, pulmonary refers to the lungs, and resucitation means to revive from a condition resembling death.

CPR RATIONALE

The reason CPR is performed is to provide oxygen to the brain, heart, and other organs until medical professionals restore normal breathing and heart action. Speed is critical. Prompt action by trained bystanders saves lives.

CPR SAFETY

Each phase of the ABCs starts with an order for assessment (e.g., determine unresponsiveness, open the airway, check breathing, check pulse). Assessment comes first, because rescue techniques that are performed unnecessarily may cause harm. It is important to remember that procedures must *not* be performed until the need has been defined.

The following techniques are to be used on infants and children from birth to 8 years of age: they should be practiced under the supervision of an instructor. During practice, do not actually perform rescue breathing or cardiac compressions on a classmate or others. These skills are to be performed on a training manikin.

AGE/SIZE DIFFERENCES

Although people come in a variety of sizes, rescue methods differ according to age. *Infant techniques* are used on those from birth to 1 year. *Child techniques* are used on those from 1 to 8 years. *Adult techniques* are used on anyone over 8 years of age.

ONE-RESCUER CPR: INFANTS AND CHILDREN

Step 1: Assessment/Airway

Assessment/airway, or the "A" of the ABCs, includes:

- evaluating the scene
- approaching the victim
- determining unresponsiveness: checking for consciousness
- opening the airway.

Evaluate the Scene

Determine if conditions are safe for you and the infant or child in need. Be aware of your surroundings. Oncoming traffic, fire, gas fumes, unsafe structures, environmental conditions, and electrical equipment can kill YOU!

Approach the Victim

Use your senses to size up the victim's condition as rapidly as possible. Look for signs of movement, signs of breathing, and abnormal positioning. Was there a fall? Could there be a head or neck injury? If so, move the victim *only if absolutely necessary,* for improper movement can cause paralysis. Look for severe bleeding. If present, have someone press on the wound to control bleeding while you continue with assessment.

Assessment: Determine Unresponsiveness

Check for consciousness. Is the child talking? Does the infant babble, coo, or cry? If so, talk quietly and in a reassuring tone and try to keep the child or infant in a resting position until ambulance personnel arrive. Never leave a child or infant alone.

The conscious infant or child who is struggling to breathe may have a partially obstructed airway. Assess breathing efforts. Apply airway obstruction techniques if indicated (see Section 5), and arrange prompt transportation to the hospital.

If the infant or child is not making any sound, position yourself at their side, tap or gently shake them, keeping in mind the possibility of a spinal injury, and ask clearly in a strong voice, "Are you OK?" If there is no response, call for help by shouting, "Help," and alert others to respond and assist. If you are truly alone, continue procedures for *1 minute* before going for help.

Position the Victim

If CPR is to be effective, the victim must be flat on his or her back on a firm, flat surface. If the victim is face down, support the head and neck and carefully turn the person face up. *Do not* allow the head to roll, twist, or tilt backwards or forwards.

Open the Airway

The *tongue* is the most common cause of airway obstruction in the unsconscious victim because the relaxed jaw allows the tongue to fall back and close over the airway. The head-tilt/chin-lift maneuver is used to elevate the tongue and open the airway. Follow these steps:

1. Place your fingers or hand on the victim's forehead.
2. Apply gentle backwards pressure (sniffing position for infants; somewhat further for children).
3. Place index and middle finger of your other hand on the bony part under the edge of the victim's chin.
4. Lift the chin upwards. Avoid closing the mouth and pressing the flesh under the chin. (Fig. 24)

Step 2: Breathing

Breathing, or the "B" of the ABCs, includes

- checking for signs of breathing
- beginning rescue breathing if the victim is in respiratory arrest.

Check Breathing: Determine Breathlessness

While maintaining an open airway, place your ear close to the victim's mouth and nose for 3 to 5 seconds and

- *Look:* can you see the chest rising?
- *Listen:* can you hear breathing?
- *Feel:* can you feel breath on your cheek?

If all answers are "Yes," then maintain an open airway and note how often the victim breaths. If all answers are "No," the victim is not breathing and is in respiratory arrest. Rescue breathing is needed.

Provide Rescue Breathing

Provide rescue breathing. Your exhaled air contains enough extra oxygen to meet the victim's needs. Begin with two ventilations. Follow these steps when providing rescue breathing for *infants* (birth to 1 year):

1. Perform head-tilt/chin-lift.
2. Take a breath.
3. Place your mouth over the infant's mouth and nose and make an airtight seal.
4. Blow slowly through infant's mouth and nose for 1 to 1.5 seconds with *just* enough force to make the chest rise. (Fig. 25)
5. Release the infant's mouth and nose.
6. Allow the infant to exhale.
7. Take another breath.
8. Blow slowly again (1 to 1.5 seconds).
9. Allow exhalation.

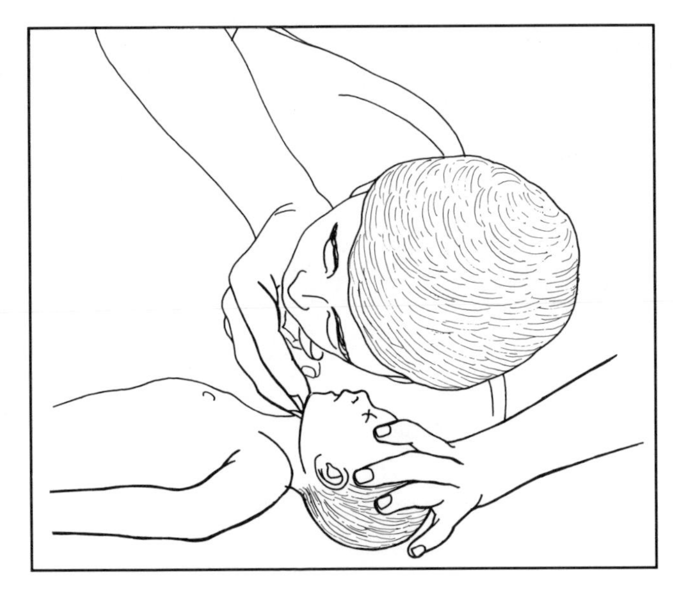

Figure 24
Head-tilt/chin-lift.

Follow these steps when providing rescue breathing for *children* (1 to 8 years):

1. Perform head-tilt/chin-lift.
2. Pinch nostrils together to prevent air from escaping.
3. Take a breath.
4. With your mouth, make an airtight seal over the child's mouth.
5. Blow slowly through the child's mouth for 1 to 1.5 seconds with *just* enough force to make the chest rise. (Fig. 26)
6. Release the child's nose and mouth.
7. Allow the child to exhale.
8. Take another breath.
9. Blow slowly again (1 to 1.5 seconds).
10. Allow exhalation.

You will know that rescue breathing is successful when you *see* the victim's chest rise and fall and when you *feel* the victim's lungs fill and empty. If breathing attempts are *not* successful, the tongue may be blocking the airway. Reopen the airway and repeat breaths. If still unsuccess-

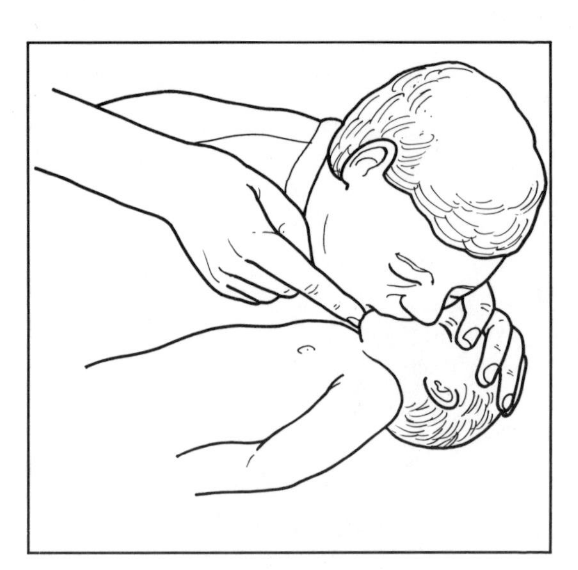

Figure 25
Rescue breathing for infants.

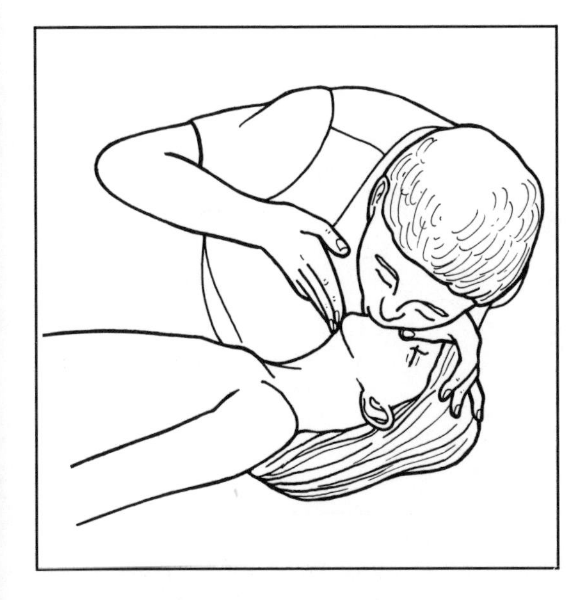

Figure 26
Rescue breathing for children.

ful, a foreign object may have lodged in the airway. Proceed with airway obstruction maneuvers (see Section 5).

Step 3: Circulation
Check Pulse: Determine Pulselessness
Circulation, or the "C" of the ABC s, includes:
- checking the pulse
- alerting the EMS system
- beginning CPR if the patient is pulseless

After providing two, full slow ventilations (1 to 1.5 seconds per inflation), check for a pulse.

Locating the Brachial Pulse on an Infant (birth to 1 year)
The infant's short, chubby neck makes finding a carotid pulse difficult. The brachial pulse, located on the inside of the upper arm, is easier to find. To locate the brachial pulse:

1. Remove clothing to expose upper arm.
2. Maintain head-tilt with one hand.
3. Place tips of your index and middle fingers on the inside, thumb on the outside, of the infant's upper arm.

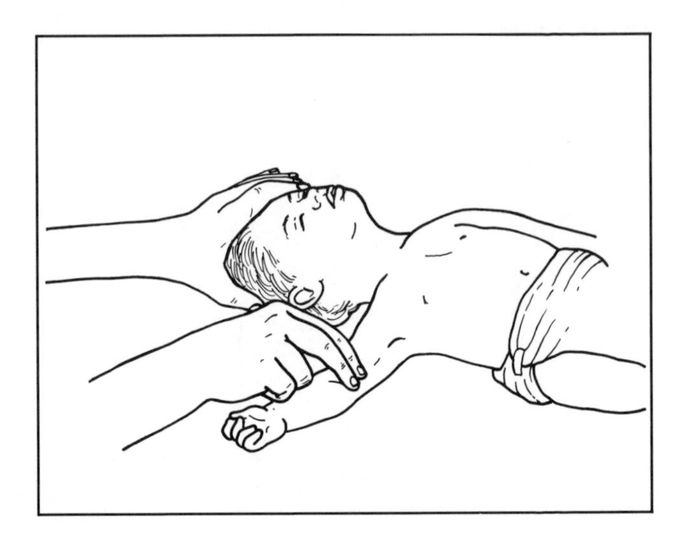

Figure 27
Locating the brachial pulse on an infant.

4. Press gently for 5 to 10 seconds to check pulse rate. Check carefully. Performing cardiac compressions on an infant with a pulse may disrupt heart rhythm. (Fig. 27)

5. Recheck breathing while check pulse.

If the pulse is *present* and the infant isn't breathing, continue rescue breathing with one breath every 3 seconds (20 times a minute). Count 1-one thousand, 2-one thousand, 3-one thousand (breathe).

If the pulse is *absent,* cardiac arrest is confirmed and both rescue breathing and cardiac compressions are needed. Make certain the infant is on a firm surface, or place head-tilt hand under baby's back and support head with your wrist and hand. A hard surface is needed to perform adequate chest compressions.

Locate the Carotid Pulse on a Child (1 to 8 year).
Carotid arteries, which are found in the neck, branch from the aorta and direct blood flow to the brain. These arteries are considered reliable because they lie close to the heart, are easily accessible, and will continue to beat after pulses

in the wrist are no longer detectable. To locate the carotid pulse:

1. Maintain head-tilt with one hand.
2. Touch victim's larynx (Adam's apple) with two or three fingers of your other hand.
3. Slide these fingers toward you into the groove between the trachea and side neck muscles.
4. Press gently for 5 to 10 seconds to check pulsebeat. (Fig. 28) Check carefully for this reason: Performing cardiac compressions on a child with a pulse may disrupt heart rhythm!
5. Check breathing at the same time you are checking the pulse.

If the pulse is *present* but the child isn't breathing, continue rescue breathing with one breath every 4 seconds (15 times a minute). Count: 1-one thousand, 2-one thousand, 3-one thousand, 4-one thousand (breathe).

If the pulse is *absent,* cardiac arrest is confirmed and both rescue breathing and cardiac compressions are needed.

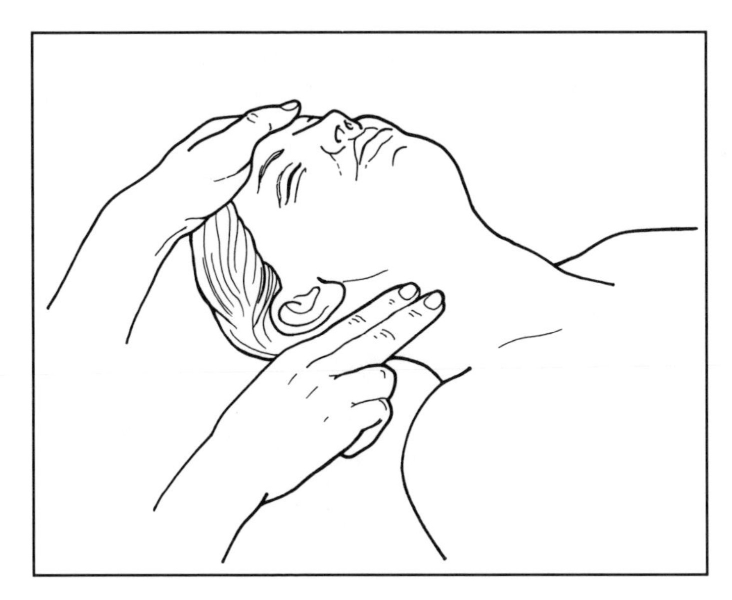

Figure 28
Locating the carotid pulse on a child.

Make certain the child is on a firm surface. A hard surface is needed to perform adequate chest compressions.

Alert EMS System

If someone arrives to help, ask that person to call the emergency telephone number and request an ambulance.

Begin CPR: Begin Chest Compressions

Studies have shown that compressions on the sternum (breast bone) squeeze the heart and increase intrathoracic pressure, creating blood flow. Rescue breathing provides the oxygen, and chest compressions provide the circulation. Chest compressions must *always* be accompanied by rescue breathing.

Proper chest compressions involve locating body landmarks and providing effective downward pressure.

Assume Proper Finger/Hand Position: For Infants (birth to 1 year)

To locate the correct landmark for performing chest compressions on an infant, follow these steps:

1. Visualize an imaginary line drawn between both nipples.
2. Place your index, middle, and ring fingers midsternum, where the sternum crosses the imaginary line.

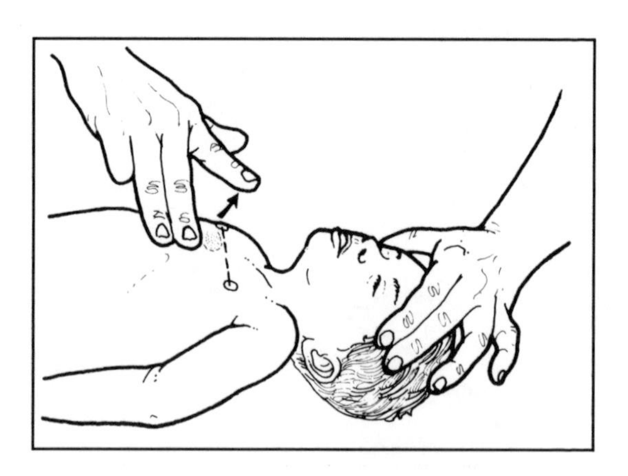

Figure 29 *Compression landmarks for infants.*

3. Lift your index finger off the infant's chest. The area of compression is beneath the middle and ring fingers. (Fig. 29)

Assume Proper Finger/Hand Position: For Children (1 to 8 years).

Kneel next to the victim's shoulders. Your upper hand (the hand closest to the child's head) will be holding the child's head in a head-tilt position. Your lower hand (the hand closest to the victim's feet) will be lying on the child's chest. To place both hands properly for CPR, follow these steps:

With your lower hand:

1. Locate the lower margin of the child's rib cage with your index and middle fingers.
2. Run your fingers up the rib cage to the middle of the chest and find the notch at the bottom of the sternum.
3. Place your middle finger in the notch.
4. Place your index finger next to your middle finger.

With your upper hand:

5. Release the head-tilt.
6. Place the heel of your hand on the long axis of the sternum next to the fingers of your other hand. (Fig. 30)
7. Remove your lower hand from the sternum because only one hand is needed for compressions on a child.

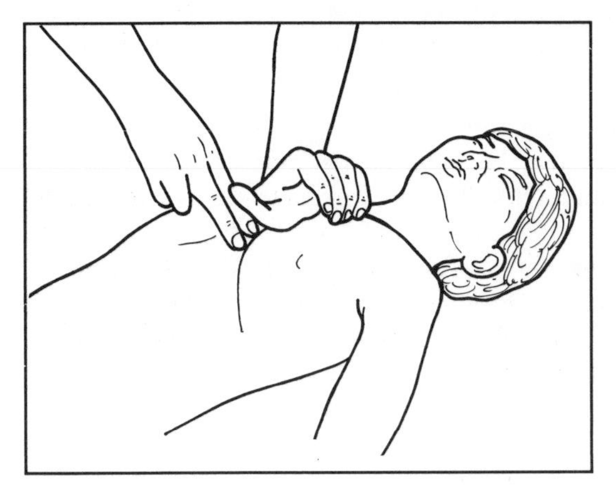

Figure 30
Compression landmarks for children.

Apply Proper Compressions

Now you are ready to begin compressions. Follow these steps:

1. Depress the sternum. For *infants,* 1/2 to 1 inch (1 to 2.5 cm) with two fingers. For *children,* press 1 to 1 1/2 inches(2.5 to 3.8 cm) with one hand. Rescuer's shoulders should be directly over the child's sternum.
2. Release the chest completely, but *do not* lift your fingers or hand from the victim's chest or correct position will be lost.
3. Compression (downstroke) and relaxation (upstroke) must be smooth and equal (50:50) to allow effective blood flow.
4. Maintain a proper rate. For *infants,* compress at least 100 times per minute (5 compressions in 3 seconds or less). Count 1, 2, 3, 4, 5 (breathe), while compressing. For *children,* compress 80 to 100 times per minute (5 compressions in 3 to 4 seconds). Count 1 and 2 and 3 and 4 and 5 (breathe) while compressing.

Step 4: Compression/Ventilation Cycles

CPR must always be accompanied by rescue breathing. To provide proper ventilations:

1. Maintain an open airway.
2. Seal the victim's mouth and nose.
3. Give one full, slow breath after 5 compressions.

Maintain proper compression and ventilation ratio (5:1). For *infants,* complete 10 cycles of 5:1 in 45 seconds or less. For *children,* complete 10 cycles of 5:1 in 60 to 87 seconds.

Step 5: Reassessment

After completing 10 compression/ventilation cycles, reassess the infant's or child's breathing and pulse to determine if spontaneous breathing and circulation have returned. Maintain open airway, and check breathing and pulse for 5 seconds. If the pulse is *present,* monitor the pulse and breathing. If breathing is *absent,* provide rescue breathing at the following rate:

1. For infants: 1 breath every 3 seconds, 20 per minute.
2. For children: 1 breath every 4 seconds, 15 per minute.

If pulse is absent, continue CPR. If no one has responded to your cries for help, it is time to interrupt rescue attempts and call for an ambulance. After contacting the emergency dispatcher, return to the victim and provide further care.

Step 6: Continue CPR
When CPR has to be continued because the patient remains pulseless after reassessment, ventilate once and resume compressions and ventilations for several minutes. Check again for the return of breathing and pulse. If absent, continue CPR.

ENTRY OF SECOND RESCUER

Transfer of CPR takes place when another CPR-trained citizen arrives on the scene. The second rescuer should:

1. Announce his or her presence by stating, "I know CPR!"
2. Call the emergency dispatcher and confirm that an ambulance is on the way by announcing that "EMS is activated!"
3. Offer assistance by asking, "Can I help?"

You, the first rescuer, decide if help is needed and if a transfer will take place. Follow these steps if you decide to let the second rescuer relieve you.

First Rescuer (you)

1. Complete CPR cycle (5 compressions and 1 ventilation).
2. Say, "Take over CPR!"

Second Rescuer

3. Moves to the victim's head.
4. Opens the airway.
5. Locates the carotid or brachial pulse site.
6. Checks pulse and breathing for 5 seconds. If breathing is absent, the second rescuer gives 1 slow, full breath. If the pulse is absent, the second rescuer starts CPR.

First Rescuer (you)

7. Monitors the patient while second rescuer performs CPR. The chest should rise during rescue breathing, and a pulse should be felt with each compression. If not, larger breaths and deeper compressions are needed.

Once ambulance personnel arrive, transfer of care occurs after the current rescuer completes a compression/ventilation cycle.

WHEN TO STOP CPR

Eventually, rescue efforts must cease. You should discontinue CPR when:

S—the victim *starts* breathing and has a pulse.

T—you *transfer* care to ambulance personnel or others trained in CPR.

O—you are *out of energy* and can no longer perform CPR.

P—a *physician* is present and assumes responsibility.

CONCERNS/ COMPLICATIONS

Problems with rescue breathing

Vomiting

Vomiting can occur at any time. The infant or child must be handled carefully, because vomitus in the lungs (aspiration) is life-threatening! Aspiration may cause a type of pneumonia that can kill the victim even after rescue efforts have been successful.

At the first sign of vomiting:

1. turn the infant/child to the side.
2. Maintain this position until vomiting ends.
3. Wipe vomit out of the victim's mouth. Use your fingers or a cloth.
4. Reposition the victim on his or her back if rescue breathing is needed.
5. Resume rescue breathing if indicated.

Gastric Distention

Gastric distention (air in the stomach) occurs when rescue breathing is performed too quickly or too forcefully, or when the infant's or child's airway is partially or completely blocked. Too much air in the stomach can cause vomiting and may limit lung expansion.

At the first sign of gastric distention

1. Reopen the infant's/child's airway.
2. Slow rescue breathing to 1 to 1 1/2 seconds per inflation.
3. Reduce ventilations. Blow just enough to make the chest rise.

If *severe* gastric distention elevates the diaphragm, limits lung expansion, and interferes with rescue breathing:

1. Turn the infant/child to the side.
2. Press their upper abdomen. Do not maintain continuous pressure because you may damage the liver.
3. Expect vomiting: when the victim has finished vomiting, wipe any vomit out of their mouth.
4. Reposition the victim on his or her back.
5. Resume rescue breathing if needed.

The unresponsive, nonbreathing and pulseless victim *must* receive a combination of rescue breathing and external chest compressions in order to survive cardiac arrest. Even though compressions will cause rib fractures and internal injuries in some victims, these injuries can be repaired after resuscitation.

To minimize injuries and provide adequate compressions:

1. Find proper landmark and *avoid* pressing over the tip of the sternum (xiphoid process).
2. With a child, elevate fingers to *avoid* pressing on ribs.
3. Evaluate depth of compression:
   - for *infants,* press 1/2 to 1 inch (1 to 2.5 cm) with 2 fingers.
   - for *children,* press 1 to 1 1/2 inches (2.5 to 3.8 cm) with 1 hand.

   Shallow compressions may be ineffective, and deeper compressions may cause injury.
4. Evaluate the type of compression: Smooth, even strokes are needed to allow heart filling. Jerky, stabbing compressions decrease blood flow.

SECTION 5: UPPER AIRWAY OBSTRUCTION IN INFANTS AND CHILDREN

CAUSES OF AIRWAY OBSTRUCTION

Causes of airway obstruction in infants and children include injuries, severe allergic reactions, infections, and obstructions from food, toys, or other foreign objects lodged in the upper airway.

Injuries

With an unconscious accident victim with possible head or spinal injury, avoid tipping the head backwards and use the chin-lift without head-tilt to open the airway. Rescue breathing should be attempted while maintaining the victim's head in a neutral position. However, if this technique does not open the airway enough to allow adequate ventilations, the victim's head must be tilted.

Severe Allergic Reaction

Severe allergic reactions are responses by the body to a specific substance (such as insect stings, food, medications, and inhaled matter). Reactions include itching, redness, hives, and swelling of the throat which can develop into upper airway obstruction. When the victim is suffering from a severe allergic reaction:

1. Assess breathing and pulse. If absent, start CPR.
2. Arrange transportation to the hospital. Special medications are needed to control reactions.

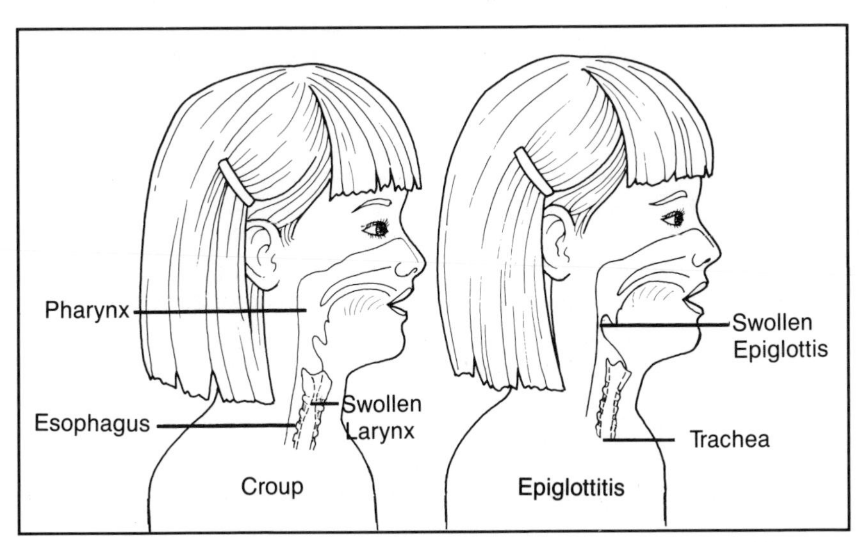

Figure 31
Croup/Epiglottitis.

Infection

Croup and epiglottitis are potentially life-threatening viral and bacterial infections usually found in children, which can result in swelling of the throat. (Fig. 31, page 77) The signs and symptoms of croup and epiglottitis include:

- fever
- breathing difficulties
- excessive, uncontrolled drooling
- high-pitched, barking cough
- the child resists lying down

Follow these steps in the emergency management of croup and epiglottitis:

1. Keep the conscious child in a seated position.
2. Be preprared to provide CPR. However, airway obstruction maneuvers are *not* to be used on victims with croup or epiglottitis.
3. *Do not put a tongue blade or finger into the victim's mouth.* This may cause the larynx (voice box) to swell shut, completely blocking the airway.
4. Arrange prompt transportation to the hospital.

Foreign Body Obstruction

Foods and small objects can lodge in the upper airway and cause breathing problems. Attempts to relieve these obstructions should be implemented when a foreign object in the airway is seen or highly suspected, or when rescue breathing attempts are unsuccessful.

RECOGNIZING FOREIGN BODY OBSTRUCTION

Objects in the upper airway may allow some airflow. Management of partial airway obstruction depends on the infant's or child's breathing efforts. Check their breathing. Is the victim displaying good or poor air exchange? With good air exchange, the child will cough forcefully and many wheeze between coughs. With poor exchange the child:

- Will cough weakly.
- Will strain to breathe.
- May make high-pitched, crowing sounds.

- May show blueness of the lips and fingernails (cyanosis).

A complete airway obstruction blocks all airflow. Recognition of complete airway obstruction depends on the child's state of consciousness. The *conscious* victim cannot cough, breathe, or cry. The child may stumble about, neck straining, while clutching his or her throat (the *universal distress signal).*

The *unconscious* victim may have visible signs of upper airway obstruction—the rescuer can see the object(s)—or the obstruction may not be discovered until rescue breathing attempts are made—the rescuer will be unable to ventilate the victim.

The following techniques are used on infants from birth to 1 year, and children from 1 to 8 years. They are to be practiced under the supervision of your instructor. During practice, do not actually perform back blows, chest thrusts, the Heimlich maneuver, finger sweeps, or rescue breathing on a classmate or others. Some of these skills may be performed on a training manikin.

MANAGEMENT OF OBSTRUCTED AIRWAY IN A CONSCIOUS INFANT

Step 1: Assessment/Airway
Evaluate the scene. Make sure conditions are safe for yourself and the infant in need.

Determine if airway obstruction exists. If the infant is forcefully coughing, resist the urge to slap the baby on the back and encourage coughing. Coughing is nature's way of clearing airway obstruction. If, however, any of the following conditions exist, action is needed:
- The infant cannot make a sound.
- Coughing efforts are weak or become ineffective.
- High-pitched noises are heard as the infant inhales.
- The lips, nails, and skin are blue.

Step 2: Back Blows

Deliver four back blows following these steps:

1. Place the infant face down on your forearm. (Fig. 32)
2. Hold the infant's jaw to support the baby's head and neck.
3. Lower the infant and forearm to your thigh, keeping the infant's head down. Gravity helps move the object out of the airway.
4. Deliver four blows between the infant's shoulder blades with the heel of your other hand, in 3 to 5 seconds. Be forceful!(Fig.32)
5. If the object is released, check breathing and arrange transportation to the hospital for additional care and evaluation.
6. If the object is *not* released, perform chest thrusts.

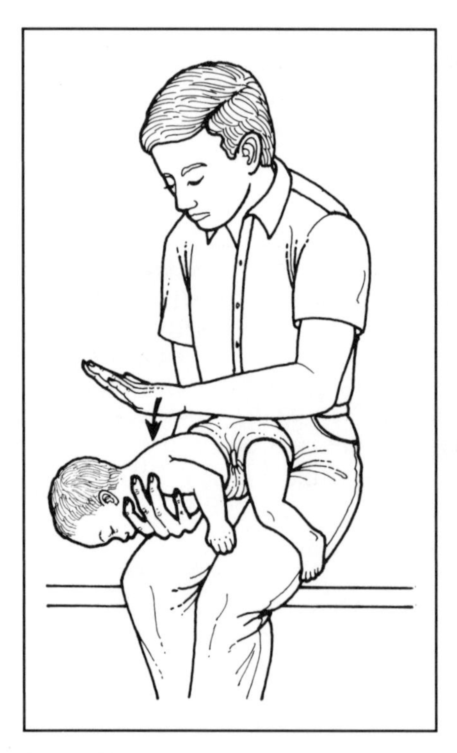

Figure 32
Back blows.

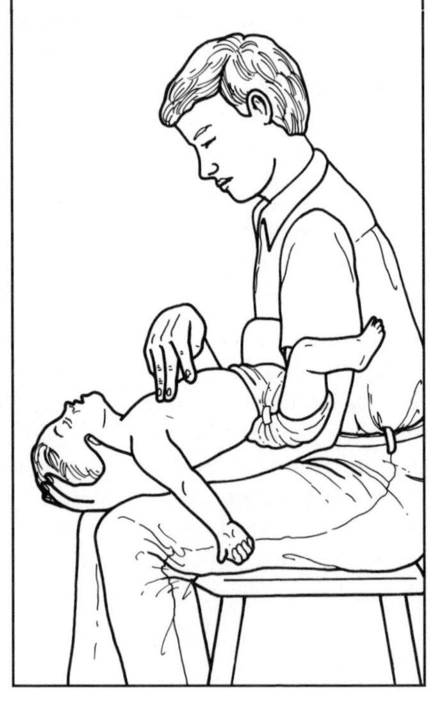

Figure 33
Chest thrusts.

Step 3: Chest Thrusts

Deliver four chest thrusts following these steps:

1. Maintain head support.
2. Sandwich the infant between your hands and forearms and turn the infant onto his or her back. Small rescuers may wish to support the infant on their lap.
3. Maintain head support while positioning the infant's head lower than their trunk.
4. Find the infant's sternum.
5. Visualize an imaginary line drawn between both nipples.
6. Place your index, middle, and ring fingers on the sternum at the intersection of the imaginary line.
7. Lift your index finger off the chest. This is the same landmark used for performing chest compression.
8. Deliver four inward thrusts within 3 to 5 seconds with your middle and ring fingers.(Fig. 33)
9. If the object is released, check breathing and transport the infant to the hospital.
10. If the object is not released, repeat back blows and chest thrusts.

Step 4: Sequencing

Repeat back blows and chest thrusts (steps 2 and 3) until the object is released or the infant becomes unconscious.

Step 5: Call for Help

Shout "Help." If someone responds, ask the person to call the emergency telephone number and request an ambulance.

Step 6: Foreign Body Check (For Unconscious Infants Only)

Open the infant's airway with the tongue-jaw lift and attempt to visualize the object. Grasp the infant's tongue and lower jaw between your thumb and index finger. Lift the jaw upward. (Fig. 34)

Look for the foreign object. If you see it, remove it with your thumb and index finger of your available hand. If the object is not in sight, *do not* attempt removal. Blind finger

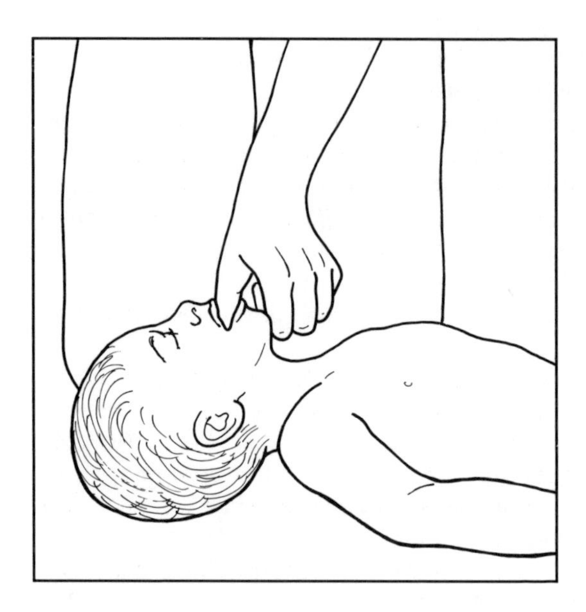

Figure 34
Tongue-jaw lift.

sweeps could push the object deeper into the airway. Attempt rescue breathing. Rescue breaths may bypass the obstruction.

Step: 7 Ventilation
Having completed a foreign body check, try ventilating the unconscious infant. Open the airway using the head-tilt/chin-lift maneuver. Seal the infant's mouth and nose and attempt rescue breathing. If successful, repeat breaths and check their pulse. Give one breath every 3 seconds, (20 per minute) until ambulance personnel take over care of the infant. If ventilations are *not* successful, deliver back blows.

Step 8: Back Blows
If the infant still does not respond after attempts at rescue breathing, deliver four more back blows. If the object is released, check breathing and pulse. If the object is *not* released, deliver chest thrusts.

Step 9: Chest Thrusts
If back blows fail to release the obstruction, deliver four more chest thrusts.

Step 10: Foreign Body Check
Using the tongue-jaw lift manuever, attempt to visualize the object. If the object is seen, remove it. Check breathing and pulse. If the object is *not* seen, attempt rescue ventilations again.

Step 11: Ventilation
Reattempt ventilations.

Step 12: Sequencing
Repeat steps 8–11 until successful or until ambulance personnel take over care of the infant.

MANAGEMENT OF OBSTRUCTED AIRWAY IN AN UNCONSCIOUS INFANT

When approaching an infant who appears unconscious, the rescuer may not realize the problem is foreign body obstruction until rescue breathing is attempted.

Step 1: Assessment/Airway

1. *Determine Unresponsiveness.* If the infant does not make a sound, tap or gently shake the baby's shoulders. If the infant does not respond. Call for help.
2. *Call for help.* Shout "Help!" and alert others to respond and assist.
3. *Position the infant.* Support the head and neck and turn the infant face upward. Place the infant on a firm, hard surface.
4. *Open the airway.* Perform the head-tilt/chin-lift maneuver.
5. *Check breathing; determine breathlessness.* While maintaining the open airway, look, listen, and feel for breathing efforts for 3 to 5 seconds. If the infant is breathing, maintain an open airway and check breath rate, quality, and depth. If the infant is *not* breathing or shows signs of poor air exchange, provide rescue breathing.

Step 2: Breathing Attempt

1. *Attempt ventilation.* While maintaining an open airway, seal the baby's mouth and nose and attempt to ventilate. If successful, give two slow, full rescue breaths (1 to 1 1/2 seconds per inflation) and check the

brachial pulse. If there is no pulse, start CPR. If rescue breathing attempts are *not* successful, the airway is blocked. Reopen the airway and ventilate again.

2. *Reattempt Ventilation.* Reposition the infant's head. Seal their mouth and nose and reattempt ventilation. If successful, check the infant's pulse. If there is no pulse, start CPR. If breathing attempt is *not* successful, activate EMS system and perform back blows.
3. *Activate EMS system.* Direct someone to call the emergency dispatcher and request an ambulance.

Step 3: Back Blows

While waiting for the ambulance, deliver four back blows;

1. Hold the infant's jaw to support their head and neck.
2. Place the infant face down on your forearm.
3. Support forearm on your thigh.
4. Deliver four forceful blows between the infant's shoulder blades in 3 to 5 seconds, using the heel of your hand.

Step 4: Chest Thrusts

If the infant is still unresponsive, deliver four chest thrusts;

1. Maintain proper head support.
2. Sandwich the infant between your forearms.
3. Turn the infant on his/her back. Keep the head lower than the trunk.
4. Deliver four chest thrusts in 3 to 5 seconds using chest compression landmarks.

Step 5: Foreign Body Check

After performing four chest thrusts, use the tongue-jaw lift maneuver and attempt to visualize the object;

1. Grasp the infant's tongue and jaw.
2. Lift their jaw upward.
3. Attempt to visualize the object. If you see it, remove it. Check breathing and pulse. If you cannot see the object, *do not* attempt removal. Try rescue breathing.

Step 6: Breathing Attempt

Attempt to ventilate the infant:

1. Perform head-tilt/chin-lift.
2. Seal infant's mouth and nose.

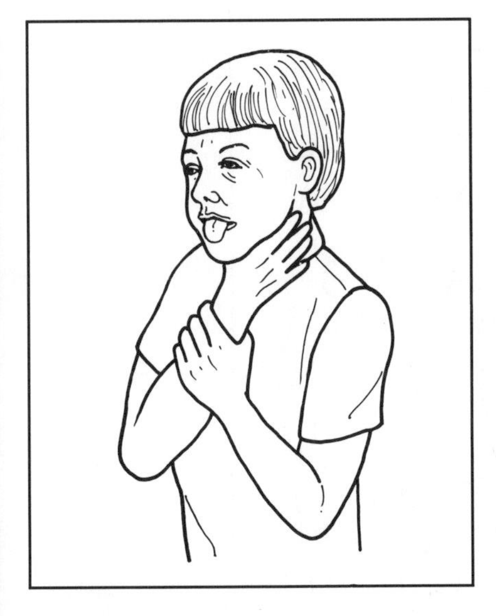

Figure 35
The universal distress signal indicating choking.

3. Attempt rescue breaths. If airway is still blocked, repeat sequence.

Step 7: Sequencing
Repeat steps 3 to 6 until successful or until ambulance personnel take over care of the infant. Remember, the lack of oxygen will cause muscles to relax. A combination of back blows, chest thrusts and rescue breathing may loosen the object, or allow rescue treating to bypass the obstruction. *Keep trying*!

MANAGEMENT OF OBSTRUCTED AIRWAY IN A CONSCIOUS CHILD

Step 1: Assessment/Airway
Evaluate the scene. Make sure conditions are safe for yourself and the child in need.

Approach the victim. Is the child staggering, neck straining, eyes open wide, and hands grasping their throat? This is the *universal distress signal* indicating choking. (Fig. 35)

Ask "Are you choking?" If the child speaks and coughs forcefully, this indicates *good air exchange*. Encourage

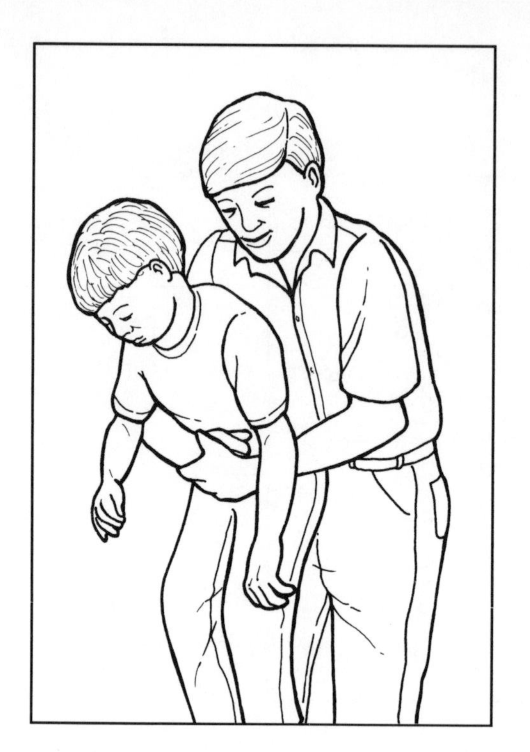

Figure 36
Abdominal thrusts (Heimlich Maneuver)—child upright.

coughing, for it is nature's way of clearing upper airway obstruction. Do avoid slapping the child on their back. Stay with the child and be prepared to help if the child develops signs of *poor air exchange* (i.e., weak cough, straining, crowing, blueness of lips, and fingernails).

If partial obstruction persists, call for an ambulance.
With poor exchange, shout "Help," and alert others to respond. Locate appropriate landmarks and perform the Heimlich maneuver.

Step 2: Heimlich Maneuver
The Heimlich maneuver, invented by Dr. Henry Heimlich, consists of abdominal thrusts which force air out of the lungs and propel the obstruction up the airway. This technique can be performed while the child is standing, sitting, or lying.

Abdominal Thrusts (Heimlich Maneuver)
When the child is standing or sitting, perform the Heimlich maneuver following these steps:

1. Stand directly behind the child.

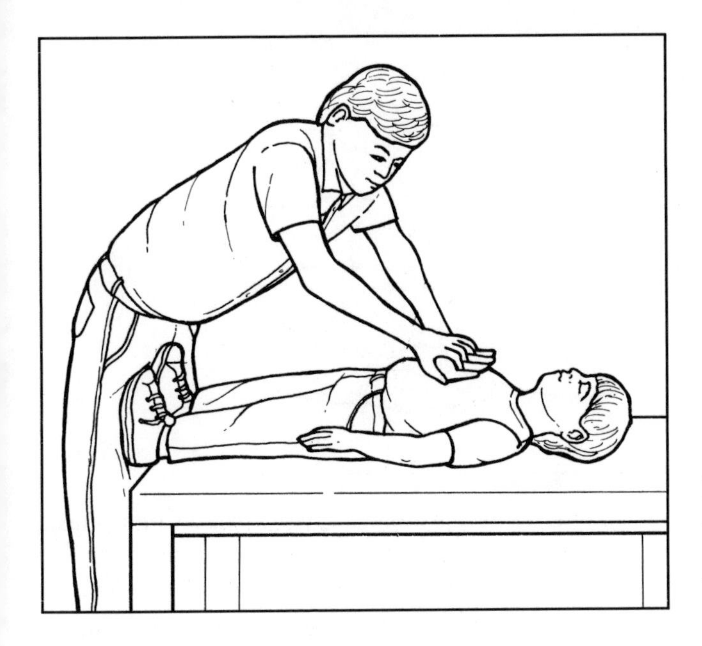

Figure 37
Abdominal thrusts (Heimlich Maneuver)—child lying.

2. Wrap your arms around the child's waist. Keep your elbows out, away from the child's ribs.
3. Make a fist with one hand. Place thumb side of your fist on child's upper abdomen, just above the navel, and well below the tip of the sternum (xiphoid process).
4. Grasp your fist with your other hand.
5. Provide swift, inward and upward thrusts until the object is released or the child becomes unconscious. (Fig. 36) Judge the force of your thrust to the size of child.

If child is lying down...
If the child has fallen but is still conscious:

1. Position the child face upward.
2. Keep the child's chin in line with their sternum. This allows proper movement of the object up the airway.
3. Kneel at child's feet if child is on the floor, or stand at child's feet if child is on a table.
4. Place the heel of your hand in the mid-abdominal area, above the navel and well below the tip of the sternum (xiphoid process).
5. Place your other hand on top of the first hand. You may interlock fingers.

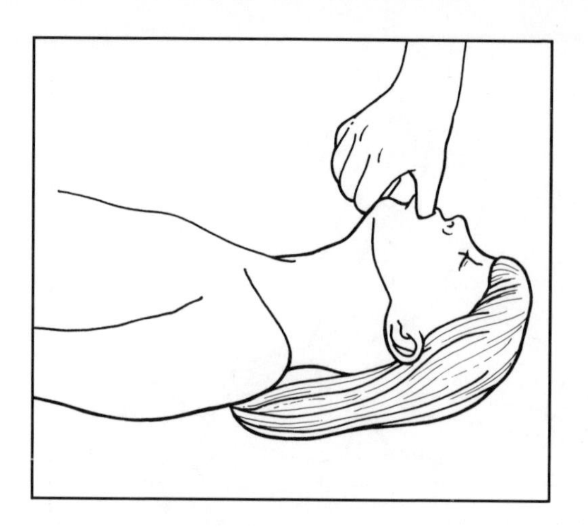

Figure 38
Tongue-jaw lift.

6. Provide swift inward and upward thrusts until object is released or child becomes unconscious. (Fig. 37) Judge the force of your thrust to size of the child.

If at anytime the child starts coughing, *Stop*! Evaluate air exchange. With *good air exchange*, monitor breathing and assure transportation to the hospital. With *poor air exchange*, continue rescue procedures.

Step 3: Additional Assessment for Child Who Becomes Unconscious

Lack of oxygen will cause unconsciousness. *Be alert*! The child can become unconscious at any time. The rescuer must be prepared to assist the victim who becomes unconscious.

Position the Victim

Do not allow the child to fall. Brace yourself and lower the child to the floor. Place the child face up, chin in line with their sternum. Do not twist the neck.

Call for help

Shout "Help"! If someone responds, direct the person to call the emergency number and request an ambulance.

Step 4: Foreign Body Check (For Unconscious Victim Only)

Open the victim's airway with the tongue-jaw lift maneuver. Grasp the child's tongue and lower jaw between your thumb and fingers. Lift the jaw upwards. (Fig. 38)

Look for the foreign object. *If you see it*, remove it with the thumb and index finger of your available hand, then check breathing and pulse.

If the object is not in sight, attempt rescue breathing.

Step 5: Ventilation
Having completed a foreign body check, try ventilating the unconscious child. Open the airway using the head-tilt/chin-lift maneuver. Attempt ventilations. If successful, provide two rescue breaths and check the pulse. If ventilations are *not* successful, perform the Heimlich maneuver.

Step 6: Heimlich Maneuver
Position the child face upward, chin in line with sternum. Kneel or stand at the child's feet and provide 6 to 10 swift inward and upward abdominal thrusts.

Step 7: Foreign Body Check
Open the airway. Grasp the child's jaw and tongue and lift upward. Remove the object if it is seen. If the object cannot be removed, try rescue breathing.

Step 8: Breathing Attempt
Attempt ventilating again. If successful provide two rescue breaths and check the carotid pulse.

Step 9: Sequencing
If after completing steps 1 to 8 you have not been able to revive the victim, begin sequencing—that is, repeat the Heimlich maneuver, foreign body check, and rescue breathing (steps 6 to 8) until the object is released and/or ambulance personnel take over care of the child. Keep in mind that lack of oxygen will cause muscles to relax. The combination of rescue procedures may loosen the object or allow ventilations to bypass the obstruction. *Keep trying*!

MANAGEMENT OF OBSTRUCTED AIRWAY IN AN UNCONSCIOUS CHILD

When approaching a child who appears to be unconscious, the rescuer may not realize the problem is foreign body obstruction until rescue breathing has been attempted and is unsuccessful.

Step 1: Assessment/Airway

1. *Evaluate the scene*. Make sure conditions are safe for you and the child in need. Approach the child. Use your senses to rapidly size up his or her condition.
2. *Determine unresponsiveness*. If the child appears unconscious, position yourself at the child's side, tap or gently shake the youngster's shoulders, keeping in mind possible spinal injury, and ask in a firm voice, "Are you OK?" If the child remains unresponsive, you many have to turn him. You must also call for help. Shout, "Help!" and alert others to respond and assist.
3. *Position the Victim*. If necessary, turn the child on to his or her back while supporting their head and neck.
4. *Open the airway*. Remember, the tongue is the most common cause of airway obstruction in the unconscious victim. Perform the head-tilt/chin-lift maneuver to open the airway.
5. *Check breathing: determine breathlessness*. While maintaining an open airway, look, listen, and feel for breathing for 3 to 5 seconds. If the child is breathing, maintain an open airway and monitor breath rate, depth, and quality. If the child isn't breathing or shows signs of poor air exchange, attempt rescue breathing.

Step 2: Breathing Attempt

1. *Attempt Ventilation*. While maintaining an open airway, provide rescue ventilations. If successful, provide two rescue breaths and check the carotid pulse. If *not* successful, the airway is blocked. Reopen the airway and ventilate again.
2. *Reattempt Ventilations*. Reposition the child's head to open their airway. Seal the child's mouth and nose. Provide rescue ventilations. If ventilations are not successful, activate EMS and perform the Heimlich maneuver.
3. *Activate EMS System*. Direct someone to call the emergency dispatcher and request an ambulance.

Step 3: Heimlich Maneuver
Perform abdominal thrusts while waiting for the ambulance:

1. Position the child face upward, chin in line with sternum.
2. Kneel or stand at the child's feet.
3. Provide 6 to 10 swift, inward and upward thrusts.

Step 4: Foreign Body Check
After performing 6 to 10 abdominal thrusts:

1. Open the airway.
2. Grasp the jaw and tongue. Lift upward.
3. Remove the object if it is seen.

Step 5: Breathing Attempt
Attempt to ventilate the child. If successful, provide two rescue breaths and check the carotid pulse. If ventilations are *not* successful, repeat procedures.

Step 6: Sequencing
Repeat the Heimlich maneuver, foreign body check, and ventilations (steps 3 to 5) until the object is released and/or ambulance personnel take over care of the child. If the unconscious child starts coughing, *stop* and evaluate air exchange. With *good air exchange*, position the child on his or her side, monitor breathing, and assure transportation to the hospital. With *poor air exchange*, repeat procedures.

CONCERNS/ COMPLICATIONS

All victims of airway obstruction must be evaluated by a physician for the following reasons:

- Foreign objects may cause bleeding and swelling.
- The Heimlich maneuver may cause internal injuries.
- Small objects may drop or be blown into the lungs.

To minimize injuries/complications:

- Assess victim carefully, and follow appropriate procedures.
- Find proper landmarks and *avoid* pressing on ribs or the tip of the sternum (xiphoid process).
- Arrange transportation of the infant or child to the hospital for additional care and evaluation.

INFANTS AND CHILDREN MODULE: QUESTIONS/ANSWERS

The following questions are based on the information found in sections 4 and 5. Circle the letter of the correct answer.

1. Popcorn is an unsafe snack for infants and small children.
   a. true
   b. false
2. Many ornamental shrubs and houseplants are poisonous.
   a. true
   b. false
3. Tap water set at 150° Fahrenheit is safe for children. It will not cause scalding.
   a. true
   b. false
4. Heart problems are the main cause of cardiac arrest in infants and children.
   a. true
   b. false
5. Rescue methods differ according to age. Infant techniques are used for those from
   a. birth to 9 months.
   b. birth to 1 year.
   c. birth to 18 months.
   d. birth to 2 years.
6. Child techniques are used for those from
   a. 9 months to 10 years.
   b. 18 months to 8 years.
   c. 1 year to 8 years.
   d. 2 years to 12 years.
7. To assess responsiveness in an infant or child who appears unconscious,
   a. shake the infant or child forcefully and slap their face.
   b. pinch the fingers and toes.
   c. place the infant or child in a face up position.
   d. tap or gently shake the infant's or child's shoulder and ask in a firm voice, "Are you OK?"

8. When rescue efforts are needed and no one else is around to help, perform procedures for one minute before leaving the victim to call for help.
   a. true
   b. false
9. The tongue is the most common cause of airway obstruction in an unconscious person.
   a. true
   b. false
10. To check breathing
    a. look, listen, and feel for ventilations.
    b. shout loudly, "Are you OK?"
    c. slap the face or shake vigorously.
    d. all of the above.
11. To provide rescue breathing for an infant,
    a. tilt the head, pinch the nose, and breathe through the infant's mouth.
    b. lift the chin, pinch the nose, and breathe through the infant's mouth.
    c. tilt the head, lift the chin, and breathe through the infant's mouth and nose.
    d. lift the chin, seal the mouth, and breathe through the infant's nose.
12. To provide rescue breathing for a child,
    a. tilt the head, pinch the nose, and breathe through the child's mouth.
    b. tilt the head, lift the chin, pinch the nose, and breathe through the child's mouth.
    c. tilt the head, lift the chin, and breathe through the child's mouth and nose.
    d. lift the chin, pinch the nose, and breathe through the child's nose and mouth.
13. When providing rescue breathing for infants and children,
    a. blow forcefully to provide maximum oxygen.
    b. blow just enough to make the chest rise.
    c. avoid blowing, since rescue ventilations, cause gastric distention.
    d. blow forcefully; infants and children need the same size breaths as adults.

14. When determining pulselessness in an infant, locate the
    a. carotid pulse.
    b. radial pulse.
    c. brachial pulse.
    d. apical pulse.
15. When determining pulselessness in a child, locate the
    a. carotid pulse.
    b. radial pulse.
    c. brachial pulse.
    d. apical pulse.
16. When the pulse is present, but the infant isn't breathing, provide rescue ventilations with
    a. 1 breath every 4 seconds.
    b. 2 breaths every 5 seconds.
    c. 1 breath every 3 seconds.
    d. 2 breaths every 6 seconds.
17. When the pulse is present, but the child isn't breathing, provide rescue ventilations with
    a. 1 breath every 4 seconds.
    b. 2 breaths every 5 seconds.
    c. 1 breath every 3 seconds.
    d. 2 breaths every 6 seconds.
18. To find compression landmarks on the infant,
    a. locate the rib margin and bottom of sternum.
    b. locate the junction of the clavicles and sternum.
    c. locate the trachea and top of sternum.
    d. imagine a line drawn between both nipples.
19. To find compression landmarks on the child,
    a. locate the rib margin and bottom of sternum.
    b. locate the junction of the clavicles and sternum.
    c. locate the trachea and top of sternum.
    d. imagine a line drawn between both nipples.
20. The compression rate for an infant is at least
    a. 60 per minute.
    b. 80 per minute.
    c. 100 per minute.
    d. 120 per minute.

21. The compression rate for a child is
    a. 60–80 per minute.
    b. 90–110 per minute.
    c. 60–100 per minute.
    d. 80–100 per minute.
22. Compression depth for an infant is
    a. $\frac{1}{4}$ to $\frac{1}{2}$ inch. (.6 to 1.3 cm.)
    b. $\frac{1}{2}$ to 1 inch. (1.3 to 2.5 cm.)
    c. 1 to $1\frac{1}{2}$ inches. (2.5 to 3.8 cm.)
    d. $1\frac{1}{2}$ to 2 inches. (3.8 to 5.0 cm.)
23. Compression depth for a child is
    a. $\frac{1}{4}$ to $\frac{1}{2}$ inch. (.6 to 1.3 cm.)
    b. $\frac{1}{2}$ to 1 inch. (1.3 to 2.5 cm.)
    c. 1 to $1\frac{1}{2}$ inches. (2.5 to 3.8 cm.)
    d. $1\frac{1}{2}$ to 2 inches. (3.8 to 5.0 cm.)
24. The ratio of compressions and ventilations for infant and child is
    a. 5:1
    b. 5:2
    c. 15:1
    d. 15:2
25. If vomiting occurs, position the patient on their side to prevent vomit from entering the lungs.
    a. true
    b. false
26. Severe gastric distention (air in the stomach) may elevate the patient's diaphragm, limit lung expansion, and interfere with rescue breathing.
    a. true
    b. false
27. Signs and symptoms of croup and epiglottitis include
    a. headache, neck stiffness, restlessness.
    b. barking cough, uncontrolled drooling, difficult breathing.
    c. abdominal pain, nausea and vomiting.
    d. bruising, pain on movement, abnormal posturing.

28. Emergency treatment for croup and epiglottitis includes
    a. using a tongue blade to view the upper airway.
    b. giving small sips of water.
    c. rapid transportation to the hospital
    d. all of the above.
29. Signs of upper airway obstruction in an infant and child include
    a. inability to cough, talk, or vocalize.
    b. high-pitched, crowing sounds.
    c. blueness of lips, nails, and skin.
    d. all of the above.
30. When performing obstructed airway techniques on an infant.
    a. position the infant face down, elevate the head, and deliver four back blows.
    b. position the infant face up, elevate the head, and deliver four abdominal thrusts.
    c. position the infant face down, lower the head, and deliver four back blows.
    d. position the infant face down, lower the head, and deliver four abdominal thrusts.
31. When performing obstructed airway techniques on a child
    a. use back blows.
    b. use chest thrusts.
    c. use the Heimlich maneuver.
    d. all of the above.
32. The tongue-jaw lift may be used in conscious victims with airway obstruction.
    a. true
    b. false
33. After performing the tongue-jaw lift on an infant or child look for a foreign object. If the object is
    a. seen, remove it.
    b. not seen, perform finger sweep.
    c. is seen, perform rescue breathing.
    d. is not seen, perform the Heimlich maneuver.

34. Rescue efforts to remove upper airway obstruction must take place even though small objects may be blown into the victim's lungs.
    a. true
    b. false

ANSWERS

1.–a	6.–c	11.–c	16.–c
2.–a	7.–d	12.–b	17.–a
3.–b	8.–a	13.–b	18.–d
4.–b	9.–a	14.–c	19.–a
5.–b	10.–a	15.–a	20.–c
21.–d	26.–a	31.–c	
22.–b	27.–b	32.–b	
23.–c	28.–c	33.–a	
24.–a	29.–d	34.–a	
25.–a	30.–c		

SECTION 6: PROFESSIONAL RESCUER/HEALTH CARE PROVIDER SUPPLEMENT

Professional rescuers (police, firefighters, first responders, emergency medical technicians, hospital employees, and others) are expected to perform the skills described in the preceding sections, as well as the two-rescuer techniques described in this section.

Two-rescuer CPR has several advantages, among them the following:

1. It is less tiring because the work of compressing and ventilating is shared.
2. The adult victim receives more ventilations because rescue ventilations are provided after every fifth compression.
3. Adequacy of compressions can be judged because the person providing ventilations can check pulses between ventilations.
4. Airways, ventilating devices (such as pocket masks, bag-valve-masks and others), monitors/defibrillators, and so forth, can be used by trained personnel to isolate and protect the airway, provide oxygen-enriched ventilations, monitor/convert heart rhythms, and give additional care for the victim by using specialized equipment.

APPROACHING THE VICTIM

Rescuers must keep in mind their own safety and approach the scene and the victim with caution. As one rescuer checks the victim and provides CPR (if indicated), the other rescuer(s) will:

1. Call for additional personnel, if needed.
2. Collect and prepare equipment.
3. Question bystanders to gather information about the incident.
4. Assist with CPR.

Additional personnel are also used for clearing the area of obstacles, moving the victim, carrying equipment, calming and controlling bystanders, and driving the ambulance.

CPR IN PROGRESS

When a second rescuer is free to assist with CPR, he or she takes position at the victim's chest, locates compression landmarks, and awaits further instruction.

The first rescuer will complete a compression/ventilation cycle (15:2), then check the victim's pulse and breathing for 5 seconds. If the pulse is *absent* , the first rescuer states, "No pulse," and gives one full, slow ventilation in 1 to 1.5 seconds.

The second rescuer starts compressions:

1. 5 compressions in 3 to 4 seconds at a rate of 80 to 100 per minute.
2. Compression depth for adult victims is 1.5 to 2 inches (3.8 to 5.0 cm).
3. Compression depth for children is 1 to 1.5 inches (2.5 to 3.8 cm) with one hand.
4. Count: One and two and three and four and five (breathe).

The first rescuer (ventilator) gives one full, slow ventilation after each set of 5 compressions (5:1, compression: ventilation ratio)—mouth-to-mask is acceptable, and will monitor compression effectiveness by checking the victim's pulse between ventilations. (Fig.39)

Figure 39
Two-rescuer CPR.

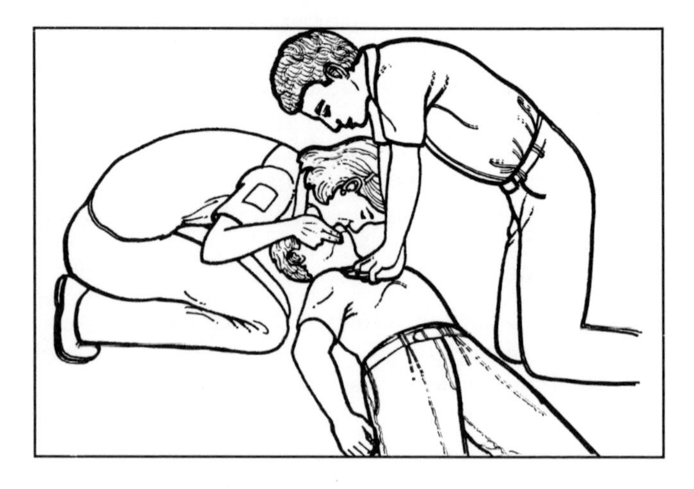

SWITCHING POSITIONS

Since the compression phase of CPR is most tiring, rescuers will want to trade places:

1. The compressor must announce his or her intentions by stating during a series of five compressions:

   "Change,
   After,
   Your,
   Next,
   Breath!"

   or state this series of five compressions:

   "Change,
   Two,
   Three,
   Four,
   Five!"

   or a similar phrase indicating the compressor wishes to switch positions.
2. The compressor completes the fifth compression.
3. The ventilator gives one full, slow ventilation then moves to the victim's chest and locates compression landmarks.
4. The compressor moves to the victim's head, opens the airway, and checks breathing and pulse for 5 seconds.
5. If pulse is *absent,* the new ventilator states "No pulse!" and gives one full, slow ventilation. These signals tell the compressor to continue CPR.

If a lay rescuer is performing CPR, professional rescuers must wait until the completion of a compression/ventilation cycle (15:2) before taking over. At that time, one professional rescuer becomes the ventilator, another professional rescuer, the compressor.

1. The ventilator checks pulse and breathing for 5 seconds. If pulse is absent, the ventilator states "No pulse!" and gives a full, slow ventilation in 1 to 1.5 seconds.
2. The compressor provides five compressions in 3 to 4 seconds for a rate of 80 to 100 per minute, and then pauses for a ventilation.

3. The ventilator provides one ventilation after the fifth compression.

Compressions and ventilations continue. Stop only for pulse checks (after the first minute of CPR, every few minutes thereafter, and when switching places), airway management or movement of the victim downstairs. CPR should *not* be interrupted for more than 7 seconds except when intubating, or at stairways.

MOVING CPR

Transferring the CPR victim from the scene to the hospital takes coordination and cooperation. Every effort should be made to move the victim carefully, without unnecessary interruption of compressions and ventilations.

Moving CPR is most efficient when the victim is transferred to a long backboard and then to the ambulance cot. (Fig. 40) Secure the victim to the board if environmental hazards (e.g., narrow hallways, winding stairs, rough ground) prevent direct transfer of the board to the cot.

When moving the victim, try to keep the patient's head and body horizontal. Tilting shifts blood flow away from the heart and brain. Position the ambulance cot at its lowest level. Higher levels are less stable and tipping may occur.

Four rescuers are involved in the transfer process. If necessary, bystanders can be directed to assist with the moving and loading procedures.

Transfer from the Scene to the Ambulance

One rescuer clears away obstacles, opens doors, carries equipment, and directs movement at stairs or slopes. Another rescuer pulls the cot from the foot end, when the passage is level, and assists in carrying the cot when necessary. The third and fourth rescuers provide CPR, using sidesteps to avoid stumbling (Fig.41).

CPR must be halted at stairways or rugged terrain. Try to keep interruptions to a minimum (no more than 30 seconds). Rescuers should pause at stair landings or level areas and provide several sets of CPR before resuming transfer.

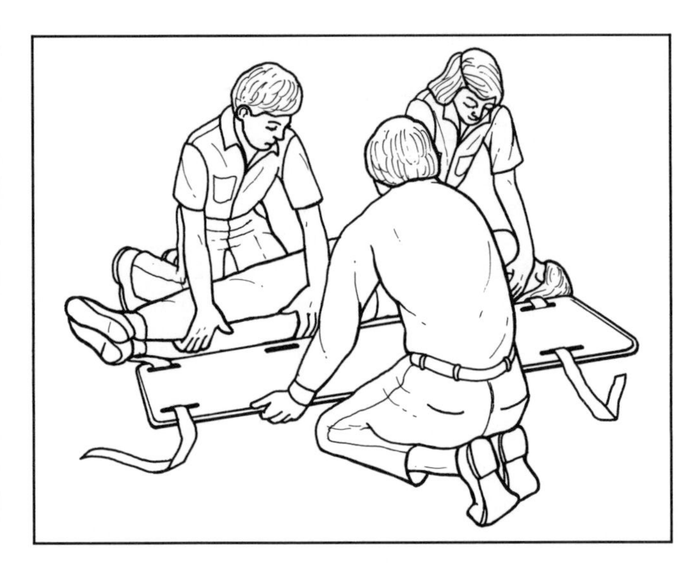

Figure 40
Place the victim on a long backboard.

Figure 41
Transfer the victim to the ambulance.

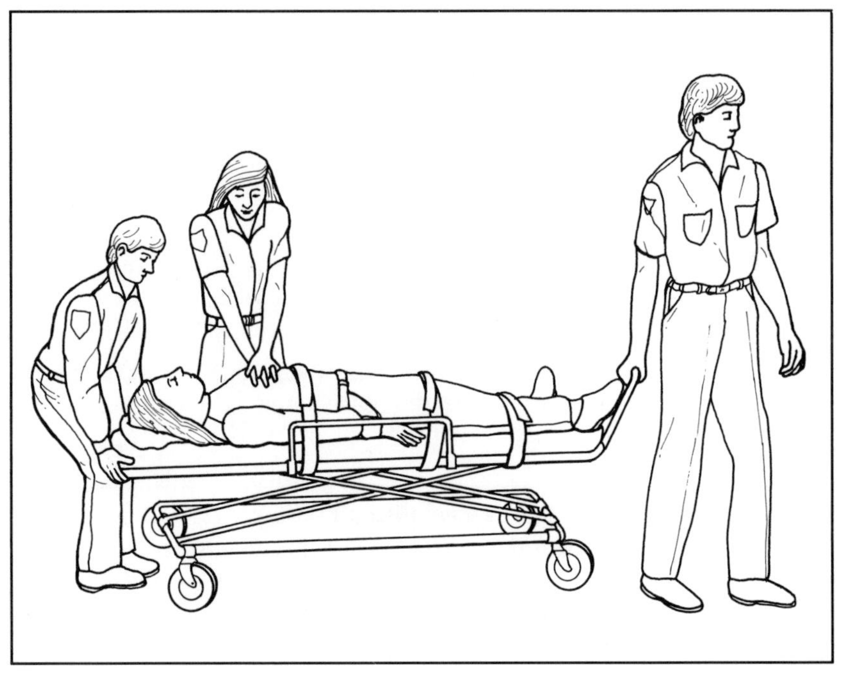

Enroute to the Hospital in the Ambulance

All rescuers assist in loading the cot into the ambulance. Once the victim is loaded, two rescuers will continue CPR.

The third rescuer stabilizes the compressor while the ambulance is moving and relieves the compressor or ventilator when either tires. The fourth rescuer secures passenger seat belts, and closes outside doors and compartments. The fourth rescuer is also the driver. The driver must follow local protocols regarding lights and sirens. The driver should also:

1. Announce out loud turns, railroad tracks, and any other road hazards.
2. Slow down at turns and bumps to provide the smoothest ride possible.
3. Communicate with the hospital regarding patient status, estimated time of arrival, and any special requests.

Upon Arrival at the Hospital

When the ambulance arrives at the hospital, the driver:

1. Opens and secures rear doors of the patient compartment.
2. Assists with unloading the victim from the ambulance.
3. Moves the ambulance to a designated parking space.
4. Secures the vehicle.

Two rescuers continue CPR until relieved by the hospital personnel. The other rescuer guides the cot to the assigned area, and provides assistance as directed by the ER staff.

After cleaning and restocking the ambulance and completing paperwork, the ambulance crew is available to accept other duties.

RESUSCITATION EQUIPMENT/THERAPY

Professional rescuers/health care providers have special equipment designed to assist rescue efforts. Never delay CPR in order to ready equipment. For the victim's sake, one rescuer must perform CPR while the others prepare gear.

If equipment is available and you have the training, the following devices may be used to:

1. visualize and remove upper airway obstruction:
   - laryngoscope
   - flashlight and tongue blade
   - Kelly clamp
   - Magill forceps
2. maintain an open airway:
   - oropharyngeal airway
   - nasopharyngeal airway
   - esophageal obturator airway
   - esophageal gastric tube airway
   - tracheal intubation
   - suction
3. deliver oxygen and rescue ventilations:
   - pocket mask
   - bag-valve-mask
   - manually triggered resuscitator/demand valve
4. record and convert heart rhythms: monitor/defibrillator,
5. provide mechanical chest compressions: automatic chest compressor,
6. correct hypovolemia:
   - intravenous infusion
   - medical antishock trousers
7. provide specific pharmacologic actions to the heart and circulation:
   - oxygen and drug therapies.

Pocket masks may be used to provide rescue ventilation during two-rescuer CPR. Mouth-to-mask breathing has several advantages, among them the following:

1. Ventilations are more pleasant.
2. If the mask is equipped with a one-way valve, there is less chance of cross-contamination.
3. If the mask has an oxygen inlet, the rescuer can provide supplemental oxygen while ventilating the victim.
4. The technique is easy to learn and often more effective than providing ventilations with a bag-valve-mask.

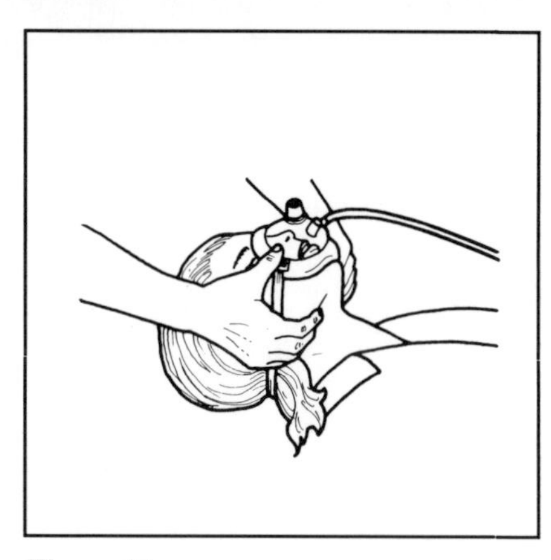

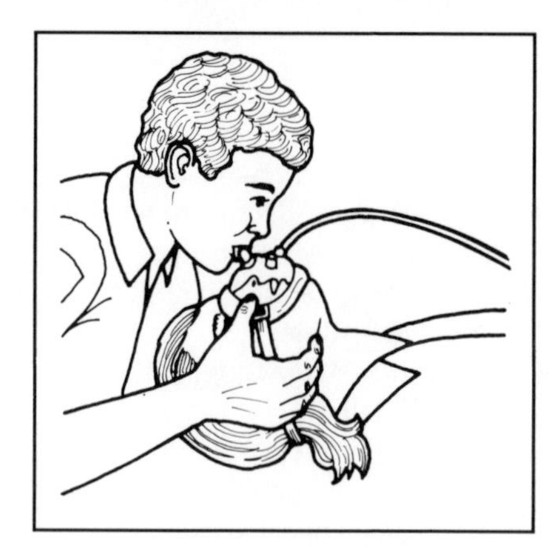

Figure 42
Using a pocket mask.
a. Spread the mask over the victim's nose and mouth.
b. Blow through the ventilation port.
c. Allow the victim to exhale.

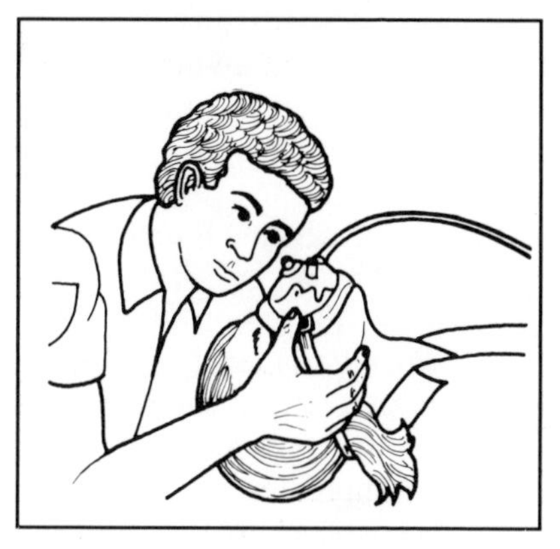

To provide rescue breathing with a pocket mask:

1. Position yourself at the top of the victim's head.
2. Spread the mask and place it on the victim's face, with the narrow end (apex) over the nose, and the wide end (base) between the victim's lower lip and chin.
3. Hold the mask firmly in place with both hands, and open the victim's airway.
   - Both thumbs are on the dome of the mask, near the ventilation port.
   - Remaining fingers are on the mask and at the angle of the victim's jaw.
   - Rest both elbows next to the victim's head.
   - Press jaw up at the angles.
4. Take a breath.
5. Seal your mouth around the ventilation port.
6. Provide one full, slow breath (1 to 1.5 seconds) with *just* enough force to make the victim's chest rise.

7. Remove your mouth from the ventilation port and allow the victim to exhale. Keep the mask in place on the victim's face. (Fig. 42)

SPECIAL SITUATIONS

Head or Spinal Injuries

For the unconscious victim with possible head or spinal injury, avoid tilting the head backwards and use the jaw-thrust maneuver to open the airway:

1. Grasp the angles of victim's jaw with index and middle fingers of both hands. Your thumb may be used to open victim's lips.
2. Rest your elbows on either side of the victim's head.
3. Lift the jaw up at the angles. (Fig. 42)

If rescue breathing is needed, seal the victim's nose with your cheek and provide mouth-to-mouth ventilations.

Trauma

If cardiac arrest is due to trauma and internal or external blood loss is suspected, control severe bleeding and use the jaw-thrust for rescue breathing, but *do not* delay transport in an effort to restore blood volume. Provide CPR and rapid transportation to the hospital. Often emergency surgery is needed to repair injuries.

Water Rescue

Float the victim onto a long backboard or other spinal immobilization device. Support the victim's head in a neutral position. Use the jaw-thrust maneuver to open the airway, and start rescue breathing as soon as safety permits. Suction may be used to clear water out of the upper airway. *Do not* use the Heimlich maneuver unless:

1. You suspect foreign matter is obstructing the airway.
2. The victim cannot be ventilated.

Check the victim's pulse carefully. People exposed to cold water are often hypothermic. Vasoconstriction and low cardiac output make assessing a pulse difficult. If CPR is indicated, make certain the victim is horizontal and on a firm surface.

PROFESSIONAL RESCUER MODULE: QUESTIONS/ANSWERS

The following questions are based on the information found in this section. Circle the letter of the correct answer.

1. With two-rescuer CPR,
   a. adequacy of compressions can be judged by the ventilator.
   b. the adult victim receives more ventilations.
   c. rescue techniques are less tiring because the rescuers can change places.
   d. all of the above.
2. Compression depth is adequate if a pulse is felt with each compression.
   a. true
   b. false
3. Compressions must be stopped to check heart action.
   a. true
   b. false
4. If during a pulse check a faint pulse is detected, continue CPR.
   a. true
   b. false
5. The signal to resume compressions is to state "No pulse," and give one full, slow ventilation.
   a. true
   b. false
6. The ratio of compressions and ventilations in two-rescuer CPR is
   a. 15:2
   b. 15:1
   c. 5:1
   d. 5:2
7. When changing positions, the ventilator announces the change.
   a. true
   b. false

8. When comparing compression rates of single-rescuer and two-rescuer CPR, it can be said that
   a. the single-rescuer rate is faster.
   b. the two-rescuer rate is slower.
   c. both rates are the same.
   d. none of the above.
9. The ambulance cot provides a firm surface for cardiac compressions.
   a. true
   b. false
10. If the victim is found in an upstairs bedroom CPR may be suspended completely while transferring the victim from the scene to the door of the ambulance.
    a. true
    b. false
11. CPR should be halted for no more than 60 seconds while moving the victim.
    a. true
    b. false
12. Moving CPR is most efficient if the ambulance cot is positioned at its highest level.
    a. true
    b. false
13. Some pocket masks may be used to provide supplemental oxygen.
    a. true
    b. false
14. With the unconscious trauma victim, perform the head-tilt and jaw-thrust to open the airway.
    a. true
    b. false

ANSWERS

1.–d	6.–c	10.–b
2.–a	7.–b	11.–b
3.–a	8.–c	12.–b
4.–b	9.–b	13.–a
5.–a		14.–b

About the Author

Barbara Trefz's interest in emergency preparation began in the 1950s, when homeowners were urged to maintain shelters for protection from natural or manmade disasters. As a youngster, Barbara stocked a basement shelter, and took Red Cross first aid and water safety courses.

The 1960s brought many changes. Although a graduate of the University of Wisconsin, Barbara for many years was a stay-at-home wife and mother. She was a self-proclaimed "professional volunteer", donating her time to church work, Jaycettes, a nursing home, school, Scouts, and the State Historical Society.

In 1977, Barbara's community asked interested residents to take Emergency Medical Technician training to provide licensed personnel for a proposed ambulance service. While enrolled in the EMT course, Barbara was appointed charter Director of Shorewood Hills Emergency Medical Service, a position she held for three years.

Barbara has been an American Heart Association Basic Life Support Instructor since 1978. In 1979 she became an employee of Methodist Hospital, Madison, Wisconsin, where she serves as Emergency Medical Services Coordinator, teaching the public, and training EMTs. Barbara has attended courses at the National Fire Academy, at National EMT Association annual conferences, and she serves as a consultant for the David Clark Company, Worcester, Massachusetts. Barbara's first published project was a handbook designed for the public, and written for the hospital, entitled "Emergency Care."

Barbara maintains memberships in the National Association of Emergency Medical Technicians, NAEMT Society of Instructor/Coordinators, the Wisconsin EMT Association, the National Registry of EMTs, ASTM and Fitch-Rona Emergency Medical Service, where she takes ambulance duty as an EMT-Intermediate.

Barbara's personal interests include her three sons, current movies, historical fiction, needlework, home decorating, travel, writing, teaching, and public speaking. Her goal is to increase public awareness of their role in emergency care.

QUICK CHECK CHART

(Adult) over 8 yrs.	(Child) 1 to 8 yrs.	(Infant) birth to 1 year

CPR

ASSESS CONSCIOUSNESS

Adult: "Are you O.K.?"	Child: "Are you O.K.?"	Infant: gentle taps

CALL "HELP!"

OPEN AIRWAY: HEAD-TILT/CHIN-LIFT

CHECK BREATHING

GIVE TWO BREATHS

Adult: pinch nose/ seal mouth.	Child: pinch nose/ seal mouth.	Infant: seal nose and mouth.

CHECK PULSE

Adult: Carotid	Child: Carotid	Infant: Brachial

ACTIVATE EMS

PERFORM COMPRESSIONS

Adult	Child	Infant
2 hands	1 hand	fingers
1½–"2"	1"–1½"	½–"1"
80–100/minute	80–100/minute	100+/minute

COMPRESSIONS/VENTILATIONS

Adult: 15:2	Child: 5:1	Infant: 5:1
4 cycles	10 cycles	10 cycles

REASSESS BREATHING AND PULSE

Adult:	Child:	Infant:
Two breaths	One breath	One breath

CONTINUE COMPRESSIONS/VENTILATIONS

TWO-PERSON CPR FOR PROFESSIONAL RESCUERS:

5 COMPRESSIONS TO 1 VENTILATION FOR 10 CYCLES.

RESCUE BREATHING

Adult:	Child:	Infant:
1 every 5 seconds	1 every 4 seconds	1 every 3 seconds

OBSTRUCTED AIRWAY: CONSCIOUS VICTIM

ASSESS OBSTRUCTION

Adult:	Child:	Infant:
"Are you choking?"	"Are you choking?"	note breathing problems

RELIEVE OBSTRUCTION

Adult:	Child:	Infant:
Heimlich Maneuver	Heimlich Maneuver	4 back blows & 4 chest thrusts

OBSTRUCTED AIRWAY: UNCONSCIOUS VICTIM

ASSESS CONSCIOUSNESS

Adult: "Are you O.K.?"	Child: "Are you O.K.?"	Infant: gentle taps

CALL "HELP!"

OPEN AIRWAY: HEAD-TILT/CHIN-LIFT

CHECK BREATHING

ATTEMPT VENTILATION

REATTEMPT VENTILATION

ACTIVATE EMS

RELIEVE OBSTRUCTION

Adult:	Child:	Infant:
Heimlich Maneuver & Finger Sweep	Heimlich Maneuver & Finger Sweep if object is seen	4 back blows & 4 chest thrusts Finger Sweep if object is seen

REATTEMPT VENTILATION

REPEAT SEQUENCE